GET YOUR Oomph BACK

A Guide to Exercise
after a Cancer Diagnosis

CAROLYN GARRITT

This book is dedicated to my dad:
fit as a flea and active to the end.

GET YOUR Oomph BACK

A Guide to Exercise
after a Cancer Diagnosis

CAROLYN GARRITT

With a Foreword by Dr Jenny Wilson

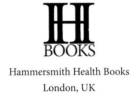

Hammersmith Health Books
London, UK

First published in 2021 by Hammersmith Health Books
– an imprint of Hammersmith Books Limited
4/4A Bloomsbury Square, London WC1A 2RP, UK
www.hammersmithbooks.co.uk

British Library Cataloguing in Publication Data: A CIP record of this book is available from the British Library.

Print ISBN 978-1-78161-211-8
Ebook ISBN 978-1-78161-212-5

Photographs: Lynn Greenfield
Commissioning editor: Georgina Bentliff
Designed and typeset by: Evolution Design & Digital Ltd, Kent, UK
Cover design by: Madeline Meckiffe
Index: Dr Laurence Errington
Production: Deborah Wehner of Moatvale Press, UK
Printed and bound by: TJ Books Limited, Padstow, Cornwall, UK

Contents

List of figures

Foreword

I initially met Carolyn two years ago at the first ever 5K Your Way Ambassadors' meeting, when she shared excitedly about her writing *Get Your Oomph Back*. Since then our contact has been a social media friendship. A few weeks ago I pre-ordered the book little expecting to hear any more about it until the published copy arrived. It was a privilege then, when Carolyn asked if, as a GP, 5K Your Way Ambassador and breast cancer survivor (13 years ago now), I would write the Foreword.

As a child I was fortunate never to have any personal experience of cancer, first learning about it as a medical student in the early '80s. I remember thinking how horrific chemotherapy seemed and wondered why anyone would choose it over quality of life for their last few months. My experience of exercise was limited too, having a lack of hand-eye co-ordination (why I am not a surgeon); I was always last to be picked for teams. I only started running as punishment, being sent cross-country running with the boys after arguing with our games teacher. I enjoyed it and intermittently carried on as the only way to exercise through the horrendous hours of a junior doctor in the late '80s.

When diagnosed with breast cancer in 2008, I was convinced I would die as a GP's experience of cancer is mainly in diagnosing, and then in palliative care, but nothing in between. I was completely unaware of the increasing number of people surviving as their care was from hospital oncology departments, and then being thrown out into the big wide world to just get on with it, without involving us. Three years before my own diagnosis, my 80-year-old mother had joined a gym to help with balance and invited me to go on a trial. I surprised myself by enjoying the strength work and so wanted to carry on exercise (albeit at home or outside rather than a germy gym) during treatment. Oncologists were shocked and discouraged me from doing weights, wanting me instead just to have a diet of broccoli and goji berries. I discovered the reality of chemo fatigue big time but found that walking (I couldn't run) was helpful both mentally and physically, so after mastectomy, against all advice, started to lift weights. The only lymphoedema I have ever suffered was after catching a blow-away marquee on Lincoln Showground.

Over the 13 years since I have been fortunate to remain well and relatively unaffected by post-cancer side effects apart from menopause. During this time the thinking about exercise and movement, post cancer but also generally, has progressed. As I have read 'Oomph' things I discovered for myself by experimentation have now become recognised. Carolyn quotes the research in her free text, particularly in the first two chapters, and references it all in an appendix. She also addresses the fact that, though statistics are important, they give none of us an individual guarantee. This is always something I struggle with. I didn't want to know my risk of recurrence as a statistic, I wanted to know would I, or would I not get a recurrence so that I could make the right (not just an informed) decision about future treatment.

In Chapter 2, Carolyn takes us through the different stages of cancer, from prehab (movement pre-treatment) to the end of life, in a compassionate, understanding and non-judgemental way. As a GP who sees patients with all sorts of medical conditions, I would also encourage all of us to move more, even before we get a diagnosis, and would encourage relatives and friends to read this book. Much of what is said is not just applicable to those with cancer but to everyone, and particularly those with chronic and long-term non-cancerous conditions. Find what you enjoy (this is crucial in order to maintain activity) and just move more. Also, to those with female genitalia (even when they have been removed), start early with pelvic floor exercises, even before any damage has been done. They are a sentence for life, and also be aware that some heavy gym exercises can cause harm. I will now get off my hobby horse!

In Chapter 3, Carolyn talks about how to get going with exercise. I had never met the concept of exercise snacks before, but realised that in our GP practice the decision to walk to the waiting room and call patients rather than use an intercom many years ago meant I was already doing this. My views on Nordic walking have changed too, now that I understand the theory behind it. I might even try it for myself one day.

Throughout the book Carolyn uses personal stories, so thank you to all those who have shared. I realised, as I was enthralled with reading, that I was becoming 'chair shaped' having been sitting too long. This caused me to move on to Chapter 4 which has all sorts of practical examples with some excellent pictorial descriptions. Fortunately no-one else was in as I found myself trying them out whilst reading in my home office.

In summary, this is a fantastic book that I wish had been around 13 years ago. As a GP I shall be recommending it to patients, and to colleagues who still don't always 'get it' when I talk about the benefits of exercise. So many need to know that parkrun does not have to involve running. I shall be recommending it to 5K Your Way attendees, though of course they are already converted. I also hope to discuss more prehab, even pre possible diagnosis for those I refer under the UK's NHS two-week rule for suspected cancer patients to be assessed.

And for me personally, when it is cold and rainy and unattractive outside, I will think of alternative ways of moving more inside.

Happy Movement.

Dr Jenny Wilson
GP, 5k Your Way Ambassador, Cancer Survivor

About the author

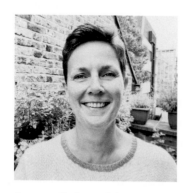

Carolyn Garritt MSc (Public Health and Health Promotion) is a cancer rehabilitation personal trainer and Exercise Lead for the West London Maggie's Cancer Support Centre. She has been working in this relatively new field for more than seven years and is a qualified personal trainer and instructor in running, boxing, sports conditioning, chair-based exercise and Nordic walking. She has trained hundreds of people recovering from or living with cancer. She also has personal experience of cancer – she helped both her parents to become more active after their cancer diagnoses and in 2020, while she was writing this book, she was diagnosed with breast cancer herself.

Acknowledgments

Professor Jane Wills, LSBU, who sowed a seed and helped it germinate.

Jenny Jen and Mr Christopher for providing a stunning space for the seedling to grow.

Lynn, for bringing me sunshine.

Bernie Byrne and Tina Glynn for their faith at the very start that it would *actually* grow, Sinead, Louise and all the team at Maggie's West London for their generous nurturing.

Huge thanks to my clients from whom I have learnt so blooming much. I am very grateful to everybody who has allowed me to tell their stories.

Particular thanks to Ren for initial direction, Chloe for reading, and Cindy, Deedee, Jane, Janet, Odile, Michelle and Vicky for listening so patiently.

Thanks too to Lynn Greenfield for her excellent photographs.

Introduction

I remember clearly the first time I heard the term 'cancer survivor' being properly described. It was in 2008 and Macmillan Cancer Support had published a report called *Two million reasons*. I listened to a presentation about it by Professor Sir Mike Richards, NHS Cancer Tsar, and one of my career heroes. He spoke eloquently and thoughtfully about some of the realities for the two million people living in the UK who had had a cancer diagnosis.

I had never really thought about what it was like to live with the consequences of cancer treatment – physical, mental *and* emotional. As I listened, I wondered why I hadn't had this awareness already. I'd known loads of things about diagnosis, and a fair bit about what treatment entailed through working in the NHS cancer screening programmes, but what happened after treatment was something that I just hadn't appreciated. That day, for me, a massive penny dropped.

Two million reasons described the broad impacts of living with and beyond cancer, and the wide range of unmet needs being experienced by people every day. It described the human perspective, rather than the clinical/medical one. At the time, cancer survival rates were increasing, but they weren't good enough; the UK lagged behind other comparable countries. The report explained that, although people did survive cancer, their quality of life was often impacted significantly. They experienced poorer health and wellbeing than the general population. The reasons why were complex and multi-faceted.

The report made a totally credible, logical argument for service provision to change and to develop swiftly, in order to better serve the growing population of people who were living with and beyond cancer. It also predicted that, with rising cancer prevalence, increased awareness of symptoms, earlier diagnosis and ever improving treatment options, the number of survivors would double to four million by 2030.

Fast forward more than 13 years and much has changed. The realities of the consequences of cancer are more broadly understood and better supported – although there's still a great deal of room for continued improvement, particularly for those living with advanced cancer. Some of the services I was offered during my own cancer treatment were the result of Macmillan's earlier clarion call.

In the field that I work in, cancer and exercise, scientific evidence now abounds, and we understand a great deal more about how exercise can help. Many organisations provide specialist physical activity classes for people with a cancer diagnosis, and there is a growing army of cancer-specialist exercise instructors on hand to help.

The scientific evidence and working knowledge are being shared widely, and people living with and beyond cancer are increasingly aware of the role that exercise might play in their future.

Sometimes, however, what's still not so apparent is 'how'. How, before, during and after the rigours of cancer treatment can we actually find the confidence, the energy and the time to be more active? What's safe? What will work? How much do we need to do?

How to use this book

This book is intended to support those who want to increase their understanding of 'why', and it hopefully explains the tremendous value of being active after a cancer diagnosis. It also shows readers 'how'.

Chapter 1 describes how physical activity can help lessen the impact on our daily lives of some of the most commonly experienced consequences of cancer treatment.

Chapter 2 looks at exercise during the various phases of cancer treatment and beyond. As you are contemplating a more active life, I urge you to be gentle with yourself – comparison can be the thief of joy after all. If you feel you are not as active, or fit, as you were before your diagnosis then do, please, acknowledge that you are in the midst of a very difficult time.

Chapters 3 and 4 become more practical and are where we start to put together plans of what to do. These 'how to' sections are intended to be useful and used often. To that end, many of the types of exercise described or suggested are ones that you can do at home, in the garden or park, either on your own or with a training buddy. (We also talk about the lovely benefits of exercising in groups, with like-minded souls.) The exercises don't require a lot of equipment and are chosen to be both safe and effective.

Chapter 3 has advice for those who are reluctant, time-strapped, tired or self-conscious – if this is you now, by all means go straight to those sections first. It's really important that the need to exercise does not start to feel overwhelming and yet another thing to try to find the energy for. Nor is it intended to suggest that 'one size fits all' – I hope the book will help you to feel in control of what you choose to do, and when. Chapter 3 contains a section on how to design your own training plan – and again, choose things that feel right for you and that matter most to you at present. Your plan will develop over time.

Chapter 4 contains sample routines which can, and should, be customised according to your preferences and abilities, which will change over time. Many of the activities can be progressed as you become fitter and stronger.

How to read the book

I suggest that you read the book through once – there will be short sections in Chapters 1 and 2 that don't apply to you, but most of it should have relevance to all.

Then go back to focus on the parts in Chapters 1 and 2 that affect you most directly, here and now, as this is the context in which you are beginning.

Then re-read the section in Chapter 3 entitled 'Do what you love', as I sincerely hope that we will find ways that you can actually *enjoy* getting your oomph back.

And then… start. The first section in Chapter 4 'Getting going' is intended to help you do just that. Look for the right level for you, now, to start to get out of puff and to start to get strong. Don't neglect the strength training: as you will come to read, it is more important than many think, and it is, I promise you, do-able.

If you can, include in your activities things that support your balance. Try to become someone who habitually does their cool down stretches. They will reduce your risk of injury and will help you keep going.

Do start small and start gently. Not wishing to quash any enthusiasm here, but I've learnt over the years that we need to spend our precious energy wisely. Aim for consistency, do little and often rather than one massive and exhausting session.

Take good rest periods – there's a section in Chapter 3 (p. 124) about active rest and recovery.

You will find after a little time that exercising becomes a bit easier and you should steadily start to feel stronger. When you reach a plateau and don't think you're improving, move on and challenge yourself a little more.

Then re-re-read 'Do what you love' in Chapter 3, to see where your ideas can take you.

The book is written for all people with cancer, and for people with all types of cancer. Often it is the most common cancers that are mentioned, partly as many of the larger works of evidence focus on them. If your particular type of cancer or treatment isn't featured, then please know that this book is still for you, and you are welcome to contact me, and I'll see what I can find to add. I have written sections about specific cancers if they tend to benefit from specific considerations or moderation when exercising, and I've written about the side effects and consequences that people have asked me about in relation to exercise.

My hope is that this book will help to empower people with a cancer diagnosis to be active and strong, on our own terms, and for the rest of our lives.

Cancer and exercise – the reasons 'why'

As outlined above, there is a growing and convincing body of evidence to describe the links between cancer and physical exercise. Much of this examines the multitude of ways in which exercise can help improve the lives, and indeed lifespan, of cancer patients and survivors.

Please note: when thinking about the links between exercise and cancer, the statistics are important, but they don't bring with them any guarantees for anybody individually; I will therefore opt for the term 'risk reduction' rather than 'prevention'.

Exercising across the whole cancer pathway

At first, exercise was only really considered, studied and suggested for people after treatment had ended. It was believed that 'rest is best' during treatment and there were concerns that exercising would be too much for the body to cope with. Increasingly though, the evidence shows that exercise can help people at every point in their cancer pathway, right from their day of diagnosis.

Cancer 'prehab', between diagnosis and the start of treatment, has been shown to have broad benefits and is being adopted across the NHS. Exercising mid-treatment – once unheard of – has been proven to be safe and to be advantageous. One clinical trial describes a chemo suite with an exercise bike in it for patients to use during their infusions.

Then, for many, comes the end of treatment – which can be a much more complex experience than many outside the world of cancer will realise. This was one of Macmillan's observations in their *Two million reasons* report – people experience a tangible sense of abandonment once their clinic visits have stopped. Many people then live with worry and 'scanxiety' during follow up or active surveillance – just ask the men undergoing regular PSA testing.

Living and exercising with secondary, or advanced, cancer is now recognised as feasible and advantageous in helping people regain a sense of control and routine during their ongoing treatment. If you follow social media, you'll find some well-known role models who are #busylivingwithcancer.

Many people probably don't realise that some hospices now have fitness suites and perhaps a swimming pool. Exercise for those in supportive care has developed significantly in recent years. It is recognised for its immensely helpful contribution to pain management and in instilling a sense of wellbeing – emotional as well as physical, even for people coming to the end of their lives.

The big picture

Exercising after cancer can save lives. Now, this is a bold statement, and, as you'll read later, I believe that we need to be cautious here because big studies of populations can give one picture but the individual stories of the people within them are myriad (i.e., it is very well established that smoking tobacco causes cancer, but most people know somebody who has smoked for all of their adult life and not developed it).

That said, evidence shows exercise can help reduce the risk of dying for people who have already had a primary cancer diagnosis. Multiple studies have shown this to be the case, and studies of the most common cancers have suggested that exercise can reduce breast, bowel and prostate cancer mortality by 30–40%.[1]

Exercise can also reduce the risk of cancer coming back and can help to slow down disease progression for people living with secondary or advanced cancer. An extensive academic review of all of the scientific knowledge in 2017 concluded that 'cancer patients involved in greater levels of exercise have a lower relative risk of cancer mortality and a lower relative risk of cancer recurrence, and they experience fewer and/or less severe treatment-related adverse effects'.[2]

Lots of us who have had cancer, or are living with it, don't know this.

What it feels like to have had cancer

Beyond the bigger picture statistics are people's everyday experiences. For many of us there are long-term health issues, often from the effects of treatment rather than the cancer itself. Sixty per cent of people who've had cancer treatment say they have unmet physical and psychological needs. If you've been through it, you may have experienced:

- fatigue
- depression, anxiety
- weight loss or gain
- altered body image
- pain, nerve damage, neuropathy
- reduced bone density, bone and joint pain
- swelling and lymphoedema
- hot flushes and night sweats.

Evidence shows that exercise can help manage **all** of these symptoms.

Is exercise the next type of cancer care?

In cardiac care, getting fit is a routine part of recovery and rehabilitation. Patients are automatically referred to specialist-led fitness classes. Cancer care services are rapidly catching up with their cardiac counterparts and there is a view that exercise may well become a fourth mode of treatment, alongside surgery, radiotherapy and chemo/biological therapies.

'If exercise was a pill, it would be prescribed to every patient'[3]

Over recent years the term 'exercise oncology' has emerged, to describe the idea that exercise could be considered a form of cancer treatment. The clarity and persuasiveness of evidence around the idea was reinforced in 2018 when the Clinical Oncology Society of Australia produced a position statement[4] that hit the headlines globally. They advised, based on scientific evidence, that exercise should be *prescribed* to all cancer patients, just like a drug. They went further than this though: they stated that exercise should be embedded as part of standard practice in cancer care, and they said that to not do so would be harmful.

Here in the UK there was some superb work in Greater Manchester to spearhead the provision of cancer 'prehab' to all people at the time of their diagnosis.[5] Prehab is now rolling out to more and more areas of cancer treatment. There are trials underway looking at exercise as a treatment option alongside chemotherapy and instead of some active surveillance in prostate cancer.

Cancer-related fatigue

Fatigue in cancer survivors is really significant – up to 95% report it. The tiredness can absolutely floor you.

Although it perhaps sounds counterintuitive, there is substantial evidence to show that exercise can help people to cope with cancer-related fatigue, and in some cases to reduce the risk of developing fatigue or lessen the severity. There are consistencies within the data – particularly in encouraging people to exercise regularly rather than occasionally and at a manageable intensity and duration. There is also evidence about the (positive) effects of higher intensity exercise.

It'll help to sort your head out

There are many psychological and emotional advantages from taking regular exercise. It can help people cope with depression, anxiety, and weariness. Running and gardening were my absolute saviours during my diagnosis and treatment.

Part of the reason that exercise can be useful here is because it can help restore appetite, thus increasing our nutritional intake, and it can help promote good sleep. Both factors, in turn, can help increase our sense of stability and our ability to cope.

As discussed later in the mental health section in Chapter 1, exercising outdoors can add further beneficial dimensions, and so-called 'green exercise' is believed to offer even greater potential support to our mental and emotional wellbeing. Part of the reason for this is that exercise helps us generate endorphins – our 'good time' hormones that can give us a happy glow.

Muscular strength, bone density, joint mobility and lymphoedema

If you've been out of action for a while, the chances are you'll have lost some of your muscular strength and this can be why simply climbing the stairs or getting out of a chair feels harder than it used to. Resistance training can help to rebuild our functional strength.

Alongside muscle loss, cancer treatments can leave us with stiff or painful joints and with a reduced range of motion, and exercise can be used to help diminish pain and to build strength in the connective tissue – the tendons and ligaments that support the joints and help them to remain mobile.

Some of the hormones used in cancer treatment are linked to lowered bone density, and there's very good evidence to show that weight-bearing exercise can help to slow down bone mineral loss and, in some cases, to actually increase bone density.

Similarly there is specific evidence that exercise, when performed with good technique, can help prevent and manage lymphoedema.

Help through transition

In this book I talk about exercising through the entire cancer 'pathway', starting at diagnosis and then onwards, for the rest of our lives. Living with cancer involves much transition from one point to the next and exercise could, in this instance, become a constant and something that is part of what we are and what we do.

It's hard to get back to work after a cancer diagnosis. Of those diagnosed in the UK, half are of working age, but cancer survivors are 1.4 times more likely to be out of work than average. Exercise increases return to work rates (although of course you may not want to go back!).

Exercise can also help you to get back to normal, to feel more like yourself or to build your own 'new normal'. It can help you get your oomph back.

Lifestyle, blame and cancer

One thing that my own cancer diagnosis taught me – starkly – is that cancer is a random lottery. Why do some of us develop it and others not? One of the reactions I often heard when I told people my news was 'but you're so fit!'. Well, as we say in Yorkshire, that's as maybe.

Despite our understanding of the statistics, it is incredibly natural to ask 'why me?' Was it luck, genes, bad timing, environmental? Who knows?

It can be perfectly possible to blame yourself, but in truth we cannot unpick our own behaviours to work out the cause.

I had a brief moment when I wondered, as a, ahem, *well-built,* gin-drinking, cake-eating, ex-smoker, how much I had contributed to my own diagnosis. Thankfully, I decided to put those thoughts away. I did grow to understand, and then make, some lifestyle changes, but I was clear in my mind that they would be positive developments, not self-admonishment.

And so I'm determined: exercise, or a lack of it, must not be used as a stick to beat people with. The same applies for body weight, body fat, BMI, diet and numerous other aspects of life that can be linked to exercise. That is simply unhelpful. What we need instead is the best information on risk reduction so that we can make our own informed choices. Self-efficacy is the aim: having the tools and methods to hand so that we can feel better and protect ourselves, on our own terms.

Exercise/physical activity/moving/fitness – what do we mean?

These terms are all broad, but in the context of this book, 'exercise' refers to any activity in which you purposefully move your body. Physical activity is defined as any movement that uses skeletal muscles and requires more energy than resting.[6] 'Exercise' is normally implied as a deliberate action, whereas 'physical activity' could occur as a result of our daily lives. You might, for example, have a job that is so physically active that you don't feel the need to exercise in your leisure time.

Exercise is often – but not exclusively – about getting a bit out of breath, doing something to deliberately raise your heart rate and make you feel a little warmer. It's also about activities that move your muscles in a way that will cause them to tire; then when they rest afterwards, they repair, and that repair process allows them to increase in strength.

A third aspect is that it might involve stretching your muscles in order to help prevent them and your joints from losing their flexibility, and it might involve activities that challenge your brain in order to restore your balance and coordination.

So, I use the terms 'exercise', 'physical activity' and 'movement' quite freely as their application to our daily lives can vary enormously. They interchange: dancing could involve a little boogie while you're cleaning with the radio on, or a full-on sweaty Zumba class. Activities such as gardening, dog-walking, picking toys up from the floor, all 'count' as exercise.

When we're thinking about becoming more active, or fitter, I would urge anyone to try to integrate into their lives these four aspects:

1. Get out of puff
2. Get stronger
3. Be flexible
4. Work on your balance.

How should it feel?

Well, it's nothing like PE at school (unless you particularly loved it, in which case you'll find there are team sports that can be accessed whether you're a beginner, a cancer patient, an older adult, or all three). It's also not about being a muscle-bound beefcake in a gym (unless that's your thing).

It definitely isn't linked to punishment, or payback for earlier life choices. And as described, it absolutely is not a reason for you to feel bad if you are not currently as active as you want to be. If this is you, please try not to feel overwhelmed. There is advice later in the book about how you can break it all down into manageable bite-sized chunks.

Being more active in this context is really about learning a broad range of options that we can choose from so that we probably feel better on a daily basis and might offset some of the consequences of treatment in the longer term.

Exercise should, however, feel like you are definitely doing something – for example, walking as exercise should not be an amble. Regardless of the speed you can reach, walking should be as purposeful and as fast as is comfortable, for you. This is because the evidence that we're using as a foundation for being more active is invariably based on 'moderate exercise' unless it states otherwise. For example, one study suggested a specific link between walking pace and cancer survival.[7] (NB the paper didn't distinguish between those who had finished treatment and those who were living with cancer.)

Exercise works best when it is an integrated part of your day, and of your life. It might take a bit of time to find that sense of integration, and hopefully this book will help with that. Exercise could and should be something that you enjoy and that you know brings you benefits.

Why we need to sit still less

A 'sedentary' lifestyle

'Sedentary' is the term used to describe a lifestyle that involves little, or no, exercise, of even the least strenuous type. It is associated with a significant risk of many health-related issues, including weight gain, obesity, diabetes and heart disease.[8]

Specifically, for those who have had a diagnosis of primary cancer, evidence shows that a sedentary life is linked to an increased risk of cancer recurrence.[9]

The term 'sedentary lifestyle' is sometimes used in a way that is derogatory, a bit 'blamey', which is not particularly helpful in the context of people who've undergone cancer treatment. That's not my intention here.

Mobility

When thinking about any desire to move more, I think it is really important to acknowledge that everybody has their own starting point. For some, the idea of increasing their levels of activity will involve running and jumping. That's fair enough, but the gains from exercise are equally pertinent to those with different levels of mobility. Your reality may well require you to spend a lot of time in a seated position, or only allow you to stay on your feet for brief spells, in which case I'm sure a lot of exercise guidance could seem completely irrelevant to you.

With that in mind, my aim is to support you to 'sit still *less*' and 'sit *less still*', rather than give the simplistic message to spend less time sitting down. We can 'sit less still' by exercising in a chair – and chair-based workouts are not exclusively gentle: some can be elevated enough to make you sweat.

Head to toe – the effects of sitting still

Many people wouldn't realise the degree to which our health is impacted by a sedentary lifestyle, beyond the big headlines above. Starting from the top, sitting still for long periods (here defined as an average of 8 hours a day) is linked to:[10]

- brain fog
- neck strain
- sore shoulders and back
- weakened chest muscles
- inflexible spine
- disk damage
- weakened abdominal muscles
- inflexible hips
- weakened glutes (the muscles in the buttocks)
- poor circulation
- reduced bone density
- varicose veins
- deep vein thrombosis
- swollen ankles.

There is a section at the beginning of Chapter 4 (p. 129) dedicated to how we can become less chair-shaped.

Chapter 1

How exercise can help with the impact and side effects of cancer treatment

Cancer-related fatigue

'Yes, that's all very well, but I'm exhausted'...

Fatigue in cancer survivors is a significant issue – it is perhaps the most common side effect. Not everyone calls it fatigue, but tiredness, exhaustion and lack of energy are reported by up to 95% of people with cancer.[1]

It varies from person to person, of course, but most people with cancer find that they have low energy. Some experience debilitating fatigue that drags on for months.

If this is you, you are not alone.

What causes cancer-related fatigue?

Well, according to Cancer Research UK, each of the main forms of treatment can cause it:[2]

- **Surgery:** people often underestimate how long it takes to get over surgery. Surgery stresses your body, and it needs time to heal. Pain can be exhausting, and the anaesthetic and other drugs may also contribute.
- **Radiotherapy:** most people who have radiotherapy feel increasingly tired as they go through their treatment. Fatigue can last for several weeks, and in some people, it can last for months after treatment has finished.
- **Chemotherapy:** nearly everyone who has chemotherapy experiences some level of fatigue, as chemo causes your white and red blood cell counts to drop midway between treatments. Knowing that you will get tired after each dose of chemo can make you feel anxious and frustrated.
- **Biological and hormone therapies:** biological drugs can cause tiredness as they can affect how your body produces the chemicals that it needs in order to work properly. Hormone treatments can disturb your body's balance and metabolism, and this can lead to many side effects, including fatigue. Drugs that block hormones in breast and prostate cancers can cause fatigue as a side effect, similar to the fatigue that women experience when going through menopause. Thyroid hormones that are used to replace hormones after surgery for thyroid cancer can cause weakness, difficulty sleeping and fatigue.

There's also the fact that being diagnosed and treated for cancer is a very big deal. It's frightening, exhausting, at times overwhelming. We sometimes don't eat or sleep or relax as much as we could or would like to, and over the weeks and months this will take its toll, emotionally and physically. I felt like I spent weeks in 'flight or fight' mode when it happened to me.

Exercise helps – but how to start?

It can be really difficult to motivate yourself to exercise when you're drained, even though it'll usually make you feel better. The trick is to start with little and often and not let the need to exercise become overwhelming. Be regular and consistent – you can always make it gentler if you need to. Work up until you can be out of breath and warm, for 30 minutes. And don't overthink – often the simplest plan is to go out for a walk. This, at times, can be enough to have a physical effect and to lift your mood, without leaving you exhausted.

Go outdoors if you can

Something that emerged clearly from the Coronavirus pandemic is people's enthusiasm for outdoor exercise. Local parks became a source of respite and escape, as well as the place to do 'Couch to 5k'. People often report a greater mood boost from going outdoors than they'd expect to feel in a gym environment. There's plenty of evidence to underpin that experience and to demonstrate that people tend to feel a sense of invigoration after exercising outdoors. One fascinating study[3] also reported that people might find exercising outdoors a little easier (i.e., their 'rate of perceived exertion' is lower doing the same activity outdoors than inside).

Exercise really can help – but how much, and how hard should you be working?

Evidence shows that exercise can be used effectively to help overcome fatigue. Much of the evidence is based on exercising at a 'moderate', level of exertion:[4] too little and it won't have as much of an impact as it could, but if you overdo it, you may end up more tired than you were when you started. Moderate exercise often entails working at 70% of your maximum heart rate.

70% MHR and its effect on fatigue

There's a scale, adjusted for age, that gauges the maximum number of beats that your heart can safely take per minute, known as your 'maximum heart rate' or MHR. It's thought that exercising at 70% of that level can be the most helpful, specifically for tackling cancer-related tiredness and fatigue.[5]

To work out your 70% MHR you use this equation:

220 minus your current age, multiplied by 70%

So, for a 60-year-old: 220-60=160 x 70%=112 beats per minute.

What does 70% feel like? It's working at a level where you're warm and you might want to take a layer of clothes off. You're breathing deeper than usual, but you can still talk in short sentences. This might, of course, sound like far too much exertion for you, especially in the early days of getting fitter. If that's the case, don't worry; just make sure that you continue to push yourself gently to work as hard as you reasonably can.

You can get all sorts of devices and gizmos that measure your heart rate, such as the Fitbit. I wear a watch that includes a built-in heart rate monitor. Some people love to have a gadget, and to measure their progress, whereas others prefer a simpler life. If this is you, see the section in Chapter 3 on how much exercise to do, and how it should feel ('The exercise prescription', p. 93).

As you walk, or indeed as you start any cardio-based exercise after cancer, try to get used to maintaining a pace where you are lightly out of puff, for as much of the walk as you can.

High intensity interval training (HIIT) and fatigue

High intensity interval training has become an extremely popular mode of exercise, and in contrast to the evidence outlined above, it has been found that exercising in short, fast bursts might be as effective as more traditional moderate exertion. A study of men recovering from testicular cancer treatment found that 'HIIT significantly improved post-intervention fatigue'.[6] Similarly, a study published the following year found HIIT to be as effective as moderate exercise in addressing fatigue.[7]

So which would I recommend? Moderate exercise, or a blast of HIIT? To be honest, whichever you think you'd enjoy most. There's an argument perhaps to start cautiously with moderate exercise, but if you're drawn to HIIT, then go for it.

The importance of strength training

There's also a really important, and often overlooked, role for strength training in overcoming fatigue. Building stronger muscles will help to make daily life –

climbing stairs, carrying shopping – feel less exhausting. Clinical studies show that a combination of cardio exercise and resistance training is your best bet in improving a sense of wellbeing after cancer.[8] Your strength training doesn't need to be complicated or time consuming: all you need to do is a routine where all your major muscles are worked against resistance. I highly recommend using resistance bands rather than weights at first – they're easy and adjustable and cheap and you're less likely to get injured with them.

To nap, or not to nap

One of the characteristics of fatigue is that a full night's sleep doesn't feel restorative enough, and you can feel a need to nap during the day. That's okay. I needed an afternoon nap, and an early night, every day after my surgery for about three weeks. I've been an enthusiastic napper ever since.

Consensus opinion seems to be that sleeping for 45–60 minutes during the day should help you get through the day without interrupting your night-time sleeping patterns.

Exercise is known to help improve sleep quality too.

Diet

There's a whole, detailed discussion to be had about the impact of nutrition on fatigue, and there is some very bad science on the subject. As is often the case with nutritional advice, good science seems to suggest your best plan is simply to have a balanced, healthy, varied diet: eat regularly, eat whole foods rather than refined, eat plenty of lean protein, plenty of fruit and veg, and keep alcohol, caffeine and sugar under control.

Mental and emotional health, depression, anxiety

Getting on with life after a cancer diagnosis is a big deal in so many ways: the shock of diagnosis, the grinding nitty gritty of treatment. There's a huge amount of adjustment that we all go through to some degree to adapt to the knowledge that, for the rest of our lives, we will be 'living with or beyond' cancer.

For many, the impact on our mental and emotional health can be multifaceted and long lasting. Macmillan Cancer Support describe the breadth of impact thus: 'It might refer to someone who is dealing with shock, distress and anxiety about what the cancer... means for them and their family. It could refer to an individual with severe depression struggling to put their life back together once treatment has finished, or someone who experiences post-traumatic stress on the anniversary of their cancer diagnosis. It also includes someone with a distinct mental health condition like schizophrenia who has just been told that they also have cancer.'[9]

You are not alone

Fear, worry, a sense of isolation, and reduced self-esteem and self-image are experienced by many, as are financial worries, sleeplessness and fatigue, which themselves can impact on our mental and emotional health. If you're experiencing any of the above, please know that you're not alone. A study by the Mental Health Foundation reported that: 'One in three people with cancer will experience a mental health problem such as depression or anxiety disorders before, during or after treatment.'[10] Similarly, the *BMJ* reports that 'depression affects up to 20%, and anxiety 10%, of patients with cancer, compared with figures of 5% and 7% … in the general population'.[11]

Alongside a growing understanding of the complexity and prevalence of mental and emotional issues arising from cancer, support is increasingly available too. Your clinical team should be able to direct you to talking therapies, possibly changes in medication, and to support groups, where you'll find people in a similar boat. I'm using cognitive behaviour therapy (CBT) to help me get my head around my fear of it coming back. Organisations such as Macmillan, Maggie's and the tumour-specific charities also have multiple sources of support and assistance.

As with all the other consequences of cancer discussed in this book, we know that physical activity can help. I wouldn't be so simplistic as to suggest that exercise will solve all this: if only it were that straightforward. However good, regular doses of activity or movement can certainly contribute to improving our mood and state of mind – both in the short and longer term.

The evidence

A huge study in the US – involving the general population rather than just people with cancer – found that exercising three to five times a week benefited mental health.[12] Looking specifically at people with cancer, a meta-analysis of 34 controlled studies on exercise and cancer noted reductions in fatigue and depression and improvements in quality of life amongst people who were physically active, with particular positive effects on psychological outcomes in those with breast cancer.[13]

One Australian study examined psychological distress in men with prostate cancer and its findings were very clear – exercise can help but its better if we get the level of intensity right: 'whether you do aerobic exercise or resistance exercise it doesn't matter, as long as it's at moderate to high intensity it's beneficial for reducing symptoms of depression and anxiety.'[14]

A much smaller-scale study found that exercise could improve the mental health of people with brain cancers.[15]

How does exercise help?

There are many psychological advantages from being active – it can help reduce feelings of anxiety, and weariness. Running and gardening did this for me.

Part of why it works is because exercise can impact upon other aspects of life that, in turn, can help support our emotional and mental health. It can help restore lost appetite, for example, and promotes good sleep.

Exercise directly affects our brain – it can improve alertness and concentration and enhance our cognitive functioning. Exercise, particularly aerobic exercise, has been shown to reduce tension in the body, and to stabilise and lift our mood. I see this with the people I train all the time – there's a sigh, they might puff out their cheeks and exhale, an 'ahhh' of accomplishment as we finish.

And then there are endorphins – chemicals in the brain, prompted by physical activity, that act as natural painkillers. They're our 'happy hormones' and they're why we often feel an emotional high after exercising. Endorphins leave you with a contented glow.

Outdoor steps

Dr Frances Goodhart is a clinical psychologist who I've worked alongside at Maggie's and is the author of *The Cancer Survivor's Companion*. She gives great advice on things that people with a cancer diagnosis can do, to help feel emotionally and mentally better, including:

- Take some gentle exercise – ideally outside in somewhere green – it is known to have an even bigger impact on mood.
- Set yourself realistic expectations; sometimes the pressure we put on ourselves is just too much. Think about what you would tell a friend and then ask why you have a different standard for yourself.
- Set yourself some goals: do some things that are kind and soothing for you.[16]

I agree with Frances that exercising outdoors can add further beneficial dimensions. I see it so often, especially with the groups I go Nordic walking with. There's certainly something about doing it with people going through something similar to you; you become kindred spirits in some regard. When people walk together outdoors, I've observed that conversations somehow seem to flow a little more readily than when you're in an enclosed space, and side-by-side with someone rather than face-to-face. It's as if people relax into it a little more. A good 'yomp' and a chat with someone who can empathise with what you're talking about is, in my experience, immensely nurturing.

If you are interested in mindfulness, I have found that making a walk more mindful can feel wonderfully uplifting. Whether you walk and take note of your body, how it moves, the sense of your socks against the soles of your feet, or whether you want to seek out different aspects of the natural world, spotting birds, trees, seeds, smells. It can make your time exercising feel all the more mentally rewarding.

Restorative yoga

As well as aerobic and resistance training, I think it's important that we make time (not always easy, I know) for some of the gentler aspects of movement. As discussed elsewhere, I love to practise yoga, although I don't teach it.

One type, known as 'restorative yoga', is especially helpful for us here, as it works on our parasympathetic nervous system, shifting us from 'fight or flight' mode to one of relaxation. Restorative yoga has proved revelatory to me because I feel very definitely but gently different after I've practised it. 'Child's pose', 'corpse', and 'legs up a wall' are examples of the gentle, slow restorative moves. I heartily recommend you try a class, ideally taught by a yoga cancer specialist.

If yoga's not your thing, tai chi and qi gong are also lovely, smooth, soothing forms of movement.

Prepare to relax.

Bone density, osteopenia and osteoporosis

I guess we rather take our bones for granted, until there's a problem. We don't tend to give much thought to what they do for us. Our skeleton supports our internal organs, protecting them and allowing them to function.

Our bones store important minerals and contain bone marrow, which is where our blood cells are made. Many people don't realise, but bones are living tissue: even after we stop gaining height in our teens, our bones constantly renew themselves to stay strong and function well.

'Bone density' relates to bone mineral content – the amount of *actual* bone that there is within our bones, if you will. After the age of 35 or so, the density of our bones naturally begins to decrease as part of the aging process. Some cancer treatments can noticeably accelerate this loss of bone density.

The higher your bone mineral content, the denser your bones are. And the denser your bones, the stronger they generally are, and the less likely they are to break.

Impact of cancer treatment on bones

There are strong links between bone health and our hormone system, and therefore certain cancer-related hormone treatments can have an impact on bone density.

This is particularly the case for breast cancer treatment in women that lowers oestrogen levels, such as chemotherapy that causes early menopause, and drugs such as Zoladex or aromatase inhibitors (anastrozole, exemestane, letrozole). Radiotherapy or surgery to the ovaries can also affect bone density.[17]

Similarly, hormone deprivation therapy in men with prostate cancer is known to cause reduced bone density.

People who had acute lymphoblastic leukaemia (ALL) as children are known to have a higher risk of reduced bone density later in life.

Osteoporosis and osteopenia

Osteoporosis, sometimes called 'bone thinning' or 'brittle bones', refers to the condition in which bones lose their mineral and bone content at a faster rate than it can be replaced.

Osteopenia is the precursor to osteoporosis in which the mineral content of bone tissue is reduced, but less severely than in osteoporosis. The main risk to people who develop osteoporosis is that they are at much greater risk of fracture.

Weight-bearing exercise

There's a great deal of evidence that exercise can noticeably help to restore bone density. Weight-bearing exercise – where you transfer your body weight from one foot to another – is particularly helpful. This is because the effect of that weight transfer is to cause jolts to the bones, and these jolts stimulate the bones into repair mode.

Understanding how weight-bearing exercise works

This is my best metaphor: imagine you're re-filling a coffee or tea caddy, or the pepper mill. If you tap the pot, the jolting causes the contents to pack down more densely. That, in essence, is how weight-bearing exercise works on your bone density – the jolting as you move stimulates your bone to pack down more tightly.

Examples of weight-bearing exercise are:
- walking, and Nordic walking
- jogging
- dancing
- playing racquet sports and golf
- climbing stairs
- tai chi and yoga.

Swimming and cycling are both excellent forms of exercise, but they are not weight-bearing. 'Weight-bearing' means we need to repeatedly make contact with the ground, while moving.

Strength matters

Having strong muscles, or building them, contributes significantly to our bone health, and our ability to move. If you consider *how* we actually move: our brain tells our muscles to pull and push our bones. The stronger and more flexible our muscles are, the more they support and move our frame.

Strength training is therefore an essential part of any fitness plan if you are trying to take care of your bones. Of course, some strength training exercises – such as walking lunges – are also weight-bearing and can therefore be doubly useful.

By far, your best bet is to combine aerobic, weight-bearing exercise (on your feet, getting out of puff) with strength training (getting strong). Schwartz *et al.* found that doing exactly this during chemotherapy helped preserve bone density in women being treated for breast cancer,[18] and Almstedt *et al.* saw similar responses in women after treatment.[19] It's the same picture for men too: those taking hormone treatments for prostate cancers have improved their bone mineral density by combining aerobic exercise with strength training.[20]

Exercise if you have already got osteoporosis

Do please check with your doctor or cancer nurse specialist if you are concerned, but frequently people with osteoporosis are advised to exercise, in order to reap the many possible benefits.

If you have osteoporosis already, it's advisable that you find ways to exercise that don't increase your risk of falling and breaking bones. Combat sports, skiing or skating are best avoided. Choose low-impact exercise, rather than activities that involve running or jumping – Nordic walking is a fantastic alternative to jogging as it gives you a good all-body workout, but with much less stress on your joints than running. Nordic walking poles can also help you to feel steadier if you're worried about falling.

Yoga and mat Pilates are also excellent forms of exercise that are both weight-bearing and muscle-strengthening. If you enjoy them, and have osteoporosis, avoid moves such as deep back bends, and moves where you bend forwards, as they can put too much strain on the spine.

Jane's story

Jane and I started training together shortly after her chemo finished. She was taking letrozole and having regular scans for osteopenia. We started with Nordic walking and resistance training and then she joined my running group for a 2–3-mile trot once a week. She soon became able to do that run quite comfortably, and then moved up to train for her first 10k.

Her first DEXA scan after she'd been running for a few months was fab – there was no decrease in her bone density. The only change she'd made in the meantime was running and strength training.

She now regularly runs parkrun and 10k races.

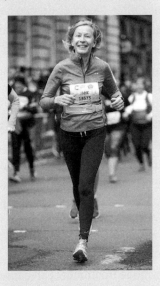

Figure 1 Jane storming towards the finish line

Weight gain, muscle loss, body fat and hormone treatments

Weight gain can be caused by chemotherapy, steroid medication and hormone therapy[21] and it is multi-faceted – it can be prompted by the onset of menopause, by changes in our metabolism and through reduced levels of exercise.[22] Muscle loss can result from reduced calorific intake, from reduced physical activity and through a slowing down of our metabolism.

Hormone treatments are used widely, long term, for people with breast, prostate and some gynaecological cancers, to help prevent cancer recurrence or to slow down disease progression. They are drugs that save lives, but the side effects can leave us vulnerable to reduced bone density, muscle loss and weight gain and increased body fat. Their effects are often felt as keenly by men as by women, and many of the consequences of the drugs are the same for both: many men will experience side effects more commonly associated with female menopause.

Now, we are definitely not going to get into 'fat-shaming' here – far from it. But one crucial aspect of exercise after a cancer diagnosis is understanding the effect that exercise can have on the composition of our bodies, particularly if they are absorbing drugs that impact our hormones. We need to consider the proportion or percentage of us that is made up of bone, muscle and fat, and how this will be influenced by treatment.

When we think of body fat, and lean muscle, many people will focus on the aesthetics, on how we look and on how our clothes fit. When we're making decisions after a cancer diagnosis, however, there's much more to consider: body composition can reduce or increase our risk of cancer coming back. Calling a spade a spade, body composition can affect our risk of dying from cancer.

Bones

It is well established that hormone treatments can cause a reduction in bone density and so, as described earlier, weight-bearing exercise is particularly helpful for people on hormone therapies.

Muscle loss

Muscle loss affects people's daily lives – it is one reason why climbing stairs and lifting shopping may feel more difficult. Many experience it as a result of spending time being less active, but it's also a consequence of weight loss caused by dietary changes. The impact on cancer patients' appetite during chemo can often lead to weight loss, as can eating difficulties for people with head and neck cancers or cancers of the digestive system. The 'weight' that is lost is often from muscle tissue as well as from body fat stores.

Also referred to as 'muscle wasting', in the short term, and during treatment, it can lead to a sense of weakness, and fatigue. It is a common side effect of hormone treatment for prostate cancer and is one of the more compelling reasons for lifelong strength training for men who've had this cancer.[23]

One condition that can arise from cancer-related weight loss is cachexia – a long-term loss of muscle that is experienced by many people, particularly those with pancreatic, gastric and oesophageal cancers. It is linked to inflammation and metabolism. Regarding muscle loss, one study recommended: 'it's important to recognise its loss and start as soon as possible preventing the development of precachexia and cachexia.'[24] Several clinical trials recommend the use of progressive strength training to reduce cachexia and the risk of it.

Measuring what we're made of

When considering our body composition, it is important to look at more than just our body weight because muscle loss can hide an increase in body fat[25] without our overall weight changing much.

Body mass index (BMI) is used widely to measure whether we are 'overweight', but it does not account for the proportion of muscle or fat in a body. It also doesn't tell us whether we are 'fit' or healthy.

Sir Chris Hoy, sprint cyclist, is currently Team GB's most decorated Olympian. He is a very muscular chap, with an incredibly powerful body. At the 2012 Olympics his BMI was 27.2, rendering him 'overweight'. The rower and multiple Olympian Sir Steve Redgrave had a BMI of 29 at his physical peak and would consequently have been considered 'obese'.

A type of weighing scale is available that will record body weight, and also an estimation of the percentage of us that is fat, water, bone and muscle mass. Basic Body Composition scales are available widely and are useful for anybody wishing to track their body fat over a period of time. They'll give you much more detail than a simple BMI measurement can. Many gyms and sports/leisure centres have fancier ones that are highly accurate.

Increased body fat – why it matters

Hormone treatments are known to increase our risk of weight gain, through an increase in body fat. This is linked to an increased risk of heart problems after prostate cancer, and a higher risk of prostate cancer recurrence.[26]

Similarly, weight gain after breast cancer treatment is really common. An oncologist I have worked with talks about 'the breast cancer stone' as she finds that's what, on average, her patients gain. Weight gain (especially more than 10% of existing body weight) is known to increase the risk of cancer mortality.[27]

I would argue that, whether we're on a hormone treatment or not, it is important that we know how much body fat we are carrying.

The American College of Exercise (ACE)[28] recommends the body fat ranges shown in Table 1. 'Essential fat' is fat that our bodies need in order to function properly. You may find it helpful to know what your percentage body fat is currently – even if you don't think that your weight has changed since your diagnosis. I found that over the course of the first year after diagnosis I gained fat around my tummy, which is typical when taking hormone medication, and I lost some muscle. Hardly a surprise, but something I'm using as a focus for improving my health and fitness in the long term. I think it would be reasonable to aim for a level that is somewhere in 'Acceptable' or 'Fitness', depending upon your natural body shape, and from your starting point today. Do please note that body fat and muscle levels change slowly. Allow yourself a period of months to work on it.

Table 1: Recommended percentage of the composition of our body that should be body fat, for women and men.

	Women	Men
Essential fat	10–13%	2–5%
Athletes	14–20%	6–13%
Fitness	21–24%	14–17%
Acceptable	25–31%	18–24%
Obesity	32%+	25%+

Cardiovascular exercise – getting out of puff – is known to encourage our bodies to use fat as fuel (often called 'fat burning exercise'). What many people don't realise is that resistance training also encourages fat burning. My absolute recommendation is that we all incorporate both into our lives, for the rest of our lives.

Moving through prostate cancer

Okay chaps, we already know that exercise is a great idea for anyone recovering from, or living with, cancer. Specifically, in men with prostate cancer, it is proven to be effective – it can help reduce the risk of cancer coming back, and for those of you living *with* prostate cancer it can help slow down disease progression.

Life after prostate treatment

I've had the privilege of training many men who've had prostate cancer treatment, and what's struck me is how their lives can be so very affected by side effects – the more common side effects of cancer treatment, such as fatigue, weakness after surgery, hair loss, weight loss or gain, and all of the physical and emotional effects of chemo.

Specifically, though, and despite maintaining a classic 'stiff upper lip' and not grumbling about it, I know that there are many men living with the impact of hormone treatment – weight gain, muscle loss, mood swings, hot flushes, tearfulness

– losing much of what can make men different from women. If you're reading this and it's sounding familiar, please know that you're not alone.

Stereotypically, men can often be more reluctant to seek support for stuff like this than women. However, being in touch with other men in the same boat as you might just help you to not feel isolated. The good people at Prostate Cancer UK can put you in touch with support.[29]

Earlier in this chapter I discussed the impact of cancer on our mental health, and we know that men who've had prostate cancer frequently experience anxiety, worry and depression as a result. Hormone treatment can impact on this significantly. My observation is that this can be heightened for those on active surveillance, and waiting for their repeated PSA test results – not easy to live with and an ongoing consequence of treatment. The section on mental health earlier in this chapter offers suggestions on how physical activity can be one of the tools available to help.

Androgen deprivation therapy, bone density and loss of strength

Hormonal therapies often used for men with advanced prostate cancer can have a detrimental effect on muscle, leading to muscle wasting. This can make you feel like you've got no strength, it can change your appearance, and everyday activities can suddenly feel much more difficult.

Another side effect of treatment can be a reduction in bone density as discussed earlier and this, plus the effect of enforced periods of inactivity, can lead to the bones becoming more brittle and prone to breakage. Weight-bearing exercise can really help here.

As well as caring for your bones, you can train your muscles to be stronger during and after prostate cancer. The secret is to start by just using the weight of your own body or light weights or resistance bands. Learn good technique so that your time will be well spent, and you minimise your risk of injury. Gradually work up to heavier weights and more repetitions.

Won't strength training increase my testosterone levels?

Good question, and one that is currently being asked by a clinical trial. One of the physiological effects of very heavy weightlifting is that it can increase your testosterone levels – which potentially could be unhelpful for men who have had prostate cancer. The current best advice is that this is only likely to be problematic in men who are doing very, very heavy lifting. Regular training is not currently believed to impact upon testosterone levels in a harmful way. Plus, the benefits of exercise far outweigh this theoretical risk.

The dreaded problem of leakage

Many men experience incontinence after treatment for prostate cancer and this can understandably affect one's confidence or willingness to get active. Don't be put off – incontinence is usually not permanent and can be helped by training your pelvic floor muscles. There's a section later in this chapter (p. 48) that explains how to do this and more details on the exercises in the first section of Chapter 4 (p. 132). The exercises can be ever so effective and may well bring a renewed sense of confidence.

Aside from training your pelvic floor, if you are worried about leakage, choose exercises that avoid bringing the knees up close to the chest, as that can squash the bladder and cause leaks. Go for moves like the pelvic tilt or glute bridge, and do squats with your feet wide apart.

In Chapter 4 you will find information specifically on how to train without squashing your belly (and bladder).

Lymphoedema

Lymphoedema is the term given to swelling that can occur as a result of fluid building up within our lymphatic system. This system can be disrupted by cancer surgery and/or radiotherapy, or by cancer cells that are in the lymphatic system itself. Normally our lymph nodes take waste fluids and move them on to be expelled by the body as urine; however, if these nodes have been damaged or removed through cancer treatment, the fluid can become blocked as its transport system can't work properly.

Cancer-related lymphoedema is experienced most commonly in the limbs, and is also found in the chest, back, groin, neck and face – places where our lymph nodes are normally at work. (I have a little area of it by my armpit.) Lymphoedema is considered a 'chronic condition' in that it tends to be managed rather than cured. It can be painfully debilitating at worst, uncomfortably inconvenient in its milder forms. Some cancer treatments (those that involve disruption or removal of lymph nodes) carry a lifelong risk of lymphoedema.

I have trained many people who knew they were at risk and were fearful of developing it. Those at risk may well have been advised to avoid certain activities, such as heavy lifting, contact sports (i.e., avoiding injury) and high intensity or endurance events, and other activities that can result in overheating or becoming dehydrated.

As with so many other consequences of cancer treatment, it is known that exercise can help – both in reducing people's risk of developing it and in helping to manage symptoms. Melanie Thomas, National Clinical Lead for Lymphoedema for Wales, says: 'Exercise is vital in lymphoedema management.' She recommends a whole range of activities, to support movement, breathing, strength and flexibility for those living with the condition.[30] Swimming and other water-based activities, such as aqua aerobics and walking/running in water, are reportedly very popular amongst people with lymphoedema. The water provides buoyancy so the affected area can feel less heavy, and this can make movement feel more manageable.

Three modes of exercise seem to jump out as most helpful (and safe): strength training, Nordic walking and some yoga-based stretches.

Support for those with lymphoedema

Helpfully, there is a growing body of clinical evidence around the management of lymphoedema, and there is support for those with the condition. I recommend the Lymphoedema Support Network (LSN) (lymphoma.org) as an excellent place for well-qualified, clinical advice on all forms of lymphoedema. For those with breast cancer-related lymphoedema, check out Breast Cancer Haven online (breastcancerhaven.org) and, if you're anywhere near to a Haven, go to see them. They're fab and may be able to point you towards appropriate professionals that offer manual lymphatic drainage – a type of massage that moves the fluid onwards.

If you have lymphoedema in a place that you can reach, you may find some relief by learning appropriate self-massage techniques. I follow an online tutorial by Dr Kelly Reed, an oncology-specialist physical therapist and lymphoedema guru. She has a richly-stocked YouTube channel called Cancer Rehab PT that you may find helpful.

Importantly though, if there's anything that is currently concerning you about your own symptoms, please talk to your specialist nurse, or oncologist.

So, should you exercise, and work on strength?

Emphatically, yes. It's recommended that people experiencing cancer-related lymphoedema DO exercise and DO train their affected areas to be stronger. Sorry about the shouty capital letters – but until recently the advice given was frequently to the contrary, and people with symptoms would be advised to avoid lifting completely – historically, women with breast cancer-related lymphoedema were advised to avoid lifting anything heavier than 2 lb (0.9 kg). This has proved to be not only unnecessarily cautious, but also unhelpful: getting stronger can help to manage the symptoms. Plus, avoiding lifting anything heavier than 2 lb didn't help anyone to get on with their life.

Part of the benefit of exercising, of course, is around how it can make you feel, how it can improve your mood and make daily life feel better and more manageable, both physically and mentally. With lymphoedema, exercise also helps to increase blood flow and oxygen to the muscles, which in turn helps the circulatory and lymphatic systems to do their work in processing and removing waste. So, it can help reduce the swelling so often associated with the condition.

Also, physical activity prompts our bodies to produce endorphins which the LSN recommend 'can help to overcome negative or sad feelings that often accompany lymphoedema'.

The evidence – Nordic walking, strength training and yoga/stretching for lymphoedema

As with other aspects of exercise oncology, there is a growing body of evidence to demonstrate the benefits that can be gained through exercise for those of us affected by, or at risk of, lymphoedema. My apologies to those experiencing symptoms in other areas of the body: almost all of the published empirical evidence focuses on women with breast-cancer-related lymphoedema. The knowledge that arises from such evidence is arguably applicable to everyone.

There's good evidence around the efficacy of Nordic walking: Jonsonn[31] found that swelling (in the arm) 'was significantly reduced after an 8-week programme of Nordic walking 3–5 times a week'. Di Blasio[32] went further and recommended that Nordic walking 'should be prescribed to prevent the onset and to treat light forms of upper limb lymphoedema'. My personal experience mirrors the evidence: I have mild lymphoedema, swelling that comes and goes. It is normally much less noticeable, and feels less tight, on days that I've used my Nordic poles.

Please see the section on Nordic walking in Chapter 3, and the step-by-step guide on how to start. Pay particular attention to swinging your arm and moving your fingers, as these are believed to be to actions most specific to reducing swelling.

Dr Kathryn Schmitz, Chair of the American College of Sports Medicine, has led the field in understanding the impact of strength training on lymphoedema. She challenged traditional thinking by conducting a trial in which women with lymphoedema followed a progressive weightlifting training programme.[33] Yep, weight*lifting* – heavy ones. The trial found that, contrary to some expectations, progressive weightlifting didn't make swelling worse. They also found that participants had fewer flare ups, reduced symptoms and increased strength.

Later Nelson[34] published a systematic review of lymphoedema and resistance exercise and concluded that 'breast cancer survivors can perform resistance training at high enough intensities to elicit strength gains without triggering changes to lymphoedema status. There is strong evidence that resistance exercise produces significant gains in muscular strength without provoking lymphoedema'.

A study published in the *Journal of Clinical Nursing*[35] looked into yoga, lymphoedema and wellbeing. The study concluded that: 'when safe to do so, the holistic practice of yoga may augment and provide additional benefit to current self-management and treatment practices for women with breast cancer-related lymphoedema.'

Before you start

There are, of course, some precautions to bear in mind. I know they're not the most comfortable garments, but traditionally it has been recommended that you wear your compression garment for the area that swells (sleeve, tights, vest etc.) during exercise. It's also recommended that you stay well hydrated before, during and afterwards, and that you look out for any changes in the affected area.

If you were given exercises to do by your clinical nurse specialist or oncology/surgical team, then do refer back to them to look for any specific advice that you were given personally. If you become tired while exercising, stop. It's one thing to work hard and push yourself, but another consistent message that I've found is that getting fitter after a cancer diagnosis, and especially with lymphoedema, is best done slowly, gently and progressively.

Some cautions

There are a few signs to look out for. Exercising should not be painful: if it is, stop. Check that your posture and technique were correct, and that you weren't trying to increase the amount of resistance you were using by too much, too quickly. This can, I'm afraid, be a matter of trial and error, so it is important to start light and build up over time. I don't want to make anyone anxious about doing this, but I do want to help avoid injury, so build up little by little, slowly and surely.

Avoid exercise if you have cellulitis. Avoid strength exercises if you've had surgery in the last eight weeks.

If your affected limb/area becomes heavy or more swollen quickly, or if you are experiencing pain, do seek the advice of your specialist nurse, physio or doctor.

There is a range of strength exercises for lymphoedema in the arms, legs and head and neck areas in Chapter 4.

Afterwards, do some deep, diaphragmatic breathing, drink water and, if you can, make a little time to relax. You might (literally) put your feet up for a few breaths: if you're comfortable doing it, lie on your back with your bottom near to a wall and the soles of your feet up on the wall, legs straight upwards.

Yoga for lymphoedema

Yoga can be a very helpful form of movement in many ways after a cancer diagnosis. It can feel restorative and empowering. It always makes me feel like I've pressed a 'reset' button. In relation to lymphoedema, yoga encourages good breathing, and yoga instructors are brilliant at teaching you how to breathe deeply and to synchronise breath with movement. We know that 'belly breathing' helps support the lymphatic system.

Yoga can also be highly relaxing, which again, helps support our natural transport systems. Yoga's combination of stretching, breathing and relaxation can help lymphoedema wherever it is, as it is a holistic form of exercise, affecting the whole body. Thinking beyond the exercises for the limbs and trunk, there are yoga poses for the face, neck and shoulders that may help specifically with lymphoedema around the head and neck.

Some yoga poses (such as downward-facing dog and child's pose) might be inappropriate for people with lymphoedema, depending upon the site of the swelling.

My recommendation is to practise yoga under the supervision of a cancer specialist teacher, even if you are already knowledgeable about yoga or have been practising it for a while. They can adapt yoga to make it safest and most effective, and they're really good at it.

Most cancer support centres, such as those run by Maggie's, Macmillan or Breast Cancer Haven, have yoga classes for their visitors. If there isn't a specialist teacher near to you, many now teach online. I highly recommend Vicky Fox Yoga (vickyfox-yoga.com) – she is incredibly knowledgeable, down to earth, and her voice is so soothing that you will, I promise, relax in her capable hands.

Lungs and breathing: climbing stairs

Breathlessness is one issue that many people with cancer experience. Regardless of where cancer was found, many people find that, as they progress through treatment, they notice that they become breathless more often. This can be exacerbated by a period of enforced rest, by weight gain during treatment, and by losing muscular strength, especially in the leg muscles. Feeling breathless is uncomfortable, and it can be worrying when you experience it. It can be a significant barrier to exercise, because getting out of breath just feels too unpleasant.

For those with cancer in the lungs, this is particularly the case, but yet the potential benefits of exercise are clear: there is evidence of the benefits of exercise at all stages of lung cancer treatment and beyond. One study recorded significant gains at the 'prehab' stage.[36] The American Lung Association reports that 'moderate exercise during lung cancer treatment can improve fatigue, anxiety, stress, depression, self-esteem, cardiovascular fitness, muscle strength, gastrointestinal side effects and breathing'. It can also help you build up your endurance and, as with other cancers, can help us to build sufficient resilience to cope with the rigours of treatment. If you have had lung surgery, then the fact that you've had some of the lung removed can impede your ability to breathe freely.[37]

There is some evidence that exercising with advanced lung cancer is advantageous – a review of studies available concluded that 'compared to those who did not exercise, people with (advanced) lung cancer who did exercise were fitter and had a better quality of life'.[38] Similarly, there are benefits for people with secondary cancer that has spread to the lungs (see the section in Chapter 2 on secondary cancer, page 68).

The best plan of action for anyone wishing to move more, and breathe more freely, either with lung cancer or with general breathlessness, is to work on five aspects of fitness:

- posture
- breathing techniques
- stretching
- getting out of puff
- strength.

Posture: stay tall

Regardless of all of the other factors, poor posture alone can restrict our ability to breathe freely. It is one of the consequences of sitting still for prolonged periods of time: the shoulders become rounded, and the head drops forward, causing the muscles around the chest to tighten over time. That tightening limits the ability of the rib cage to expand and causes us to take more rapid, shallow breaths.

As much as you can, try to stay tall, keeping your back long and straight (whether you're seated or standing) try to look forwards, rather than downwards. In an age where we spend so much time looking at screens, this is even more important.

Breathe deeply and rhythmically

We do it all the time of course, but we often don't do it well. So, remind yourself what good, deep breathing feels like. There are breathing exercises, and a whole section on ways to bring stair climbing into your exercise routine, in Chapter 4 (page 131).

Stretch your upper body

We know that sitting still for long periods of time can shorten the muscles around the chest, thus impeding our breathing. The Roy Castle Lung Cancer Foundation advises: 'Regular stretching exercises for your upper body will help improve mobility in your chest and back. It also helps your lungs and diaphragm move more freely, encouraging deeper breathing and improving circulation.' [39] Incidentally, if your exercise of choice is swimming, stretching your upper body can help improve both your breathing in the water, and your buoyancy.[40]

There is a full body stretch routine in Chapter 4 (page 195).

Get out of puff

Once you're confident that you can control your breathing, using the exercises in Chapter 4 (page 130), try challenging yourself to get lightly out of puff every day. Start gently and add in things like walking briskly to a given landmark. Try to walk a little bit faster or further than you did yesterday. Don't overdo it though – allow yourself to stay comfortable and in control. Try some of the ideas listed in Chapter 3 in the section on 'Active daily living and exercise "snacks"' (page 91).

Get strong

Your gluteal muscles – the big muscles in your buttocks – are your powerhouses for lifting your body. Like the chest muscles, they are affected by sitting, but rather than becoming tight, they become weaker and become less able to power us up or along. Have a look at the lower body strength moves in Chapter 4 (page 172) – they'll help. Or take a leaf out of Hima's book.

How Hima got fit for surgery

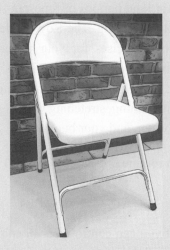

Figure 2 Hima simply used a chair

Hima was diagnosed with lung cancer and, although surgery was the best treatment option, her surgical team felt that she would find it difficult to tolerate. So, aged in her mid-eighties, she was advised to get fitter so that she could safely have her surgery. She started coming along to the gentle exercise class that I run. I don't think she had done anything like it before in her life.

At the end of each class, the whole group does as many 'sit-to-stand' exercises as they feel they can. This exercise gets you properly out of puff, sends the heart rate right up, and is helpful for building strength in your lower body and confidence in your own ability. It is the one exercise, more than any other, that I urge people to do at home as well as in the class, and Hima did her home study with considerable gusto. She just got completely into doing sit-to-stand, and would bob up and down, grinning. The number she could do increased massively over the weeks until she reached the magnificent point that she outdid everyone else in the room, keeping going longer than any of her classmates, most of whom were 20, 30, 40 years younger than her. She was able to stand up out of a chair and sit down again more than 60 times. The average for her age is nine to 14.

And then she disappeared from the class. Her family got in touch a little later to say that she had had her surgery.

Why does climbing stairs feel so tough?

Sometimes climbing the stairs can feel hard. You get out of puff, your legs feel heavy, and you need to use the banister to pull yourself up. If you're suffering from fatigue or are generally out of condition following treatment, everyday movement can feel laboured. Some people find that they become fearful about climbing steps and might go out of their way to avoid them.

It is quite normal to get out of breath on stairs, and even the fittest runners say that even though they can run for miles, they can find themselves puffing after a couple of flights. Here's the explanation: as you climb stairs, your legs must lift your body upwards, instead of just propelling it forwards. This requires extra oxygen for your legs and so your heart and lungs need to work harder to deliver it.

We often hit a staircase relatively quickly and with little run-up and so, rather than being warmed up and prepared, it's a shock to the system. And then to compound the effect, we often don't breathe effectively as we go upstairs. It's hardly a surprise then, that we start puffing and panting.

There are broad benefits in training to climb stairs in addition to the improvement in day-to-day living. Climbing up steps or stairs is weight-bearing, so you'll be improving the strength and density of your bones. It's a form of cardiovascular exercise, so you'll improve the capacity and functioning of your heart and lungs. As you elevate your heart rate, you'll burn calories as you go, and you'll improve the strength of the muscles on your lower body.

Onwards and upwards!

Exercising with an ostomy

For people undergoing treatment for colorectal, gynaecological, bladder, urinary tract or prostate cancers, one of the commonly experienced surgical procedures is the creation of a stoma. A stoma is an opening on the abdomen that can be connected to either your digestive or urinary system to allow waste (urine or faeces) to be diverted out of your body.[41] A stoma can be temporary or permanent and can be one of the physical consequences of cancer treatment that takes a while to get used to, and to accept.

If you have a stoma – or 'ostomy' – then almost all of the content of this book applies to you, particularly the parts about the benefits of exercise and of strength training, and the role of exercise in getting to grips with fatigue, which is common in those who have one.

Many people with an ostomy are, however, understandably reticent about embarking upon an exercise programme; in fact, Sarah Russell, author of the excellent *Bowel Cancer Toolkit,*[42] reports that 90% of people with a stoma say that they exercise less than is recommended for good health. Although it's completely natural to be cautious, it doesn't need to be like this.

Three issues seem to form the biggest barriers: leakage (and the fear of it), dehydration and the risk of parastomal hernia.

Dread of leakage

I have worked with many who have had a stoma at some point. I've never known one leak during exercise, although some people have worried that it might happen, especially at first.

(By the way I *have* known them make a farting noise and worked very closely with someone whose stoma was particularly noisy when she exercised. If we were out in public and it happened, she would simply and accusingly exclaim 'Oh Carolyn!', thus blaming me in the eyes of any passers-by.)

As preparation, and for reassurance, your pouch should be emptied before exercising and can be framed with waterproof tape against the skin for extra security when you move. Using skin barrier wipes also can help protect against leakage due to perspiration. Many of the pouches available now are comfortable and secure enough even for vigorous physical activity.

Dehydration

Avoiding dehydration is a consideration for anyone exercising but is particularly relevant here. My experience is that people with an ostomy – especially ileostomy – are usually well versed in the importance of staying properly hydrated. Do please bear in mind, however, that even moderate or gentle exercise can cause us to need to take on extra fluids. People with an ostomy are advised to include electrolyte drinks in their fluid intake.

Perhaps surprisingly, you also need to make sure you don't drink too much liquid during exercise as this can cause great strain on your kidneys: hyponatraemia has put paid to many marathon runners' dreams after they drank too much water on their big day. Sipping little and often is the key.

Parastomal hernia: risk

A parastomal hernia is a swelling, or bulge, around the stoma site. They occur when the edges of the stoma come away from the muscle, and this allows a section of bowel to protrude. They can cause difficulties with stoma function and they normally occur gradually over a period of time. Parastomal hernias are common, and up to 70% of people with an ostomy will develop one.[43]

People with a stoma are often very worried about developing a hernia even though, as Sarah Russell explains, they don't necessarily cause problems themselves. She says, 'Fear prevents people becoming active'.

To reduce the risk of hernia, clinical guidelines recommend some broad lifestyle changes, including maintaining a healthy body weight and not smoking. (Hernia are believed to be caused by multiple factors.) Beyond that, people with an ostomy are advised to increase the strength in their abdominal muscles, to increase their overall fitness and to use a specific breathing technique – exhale when you exert – when lifting anything at all heavy.

How to strengthen your abdominal muscles

Strength training is important in so many aspects of our lives after a cancer diagnosis, and for those with an ostomy the benefits far outweigh the risks. Normally in introducing strength training I will be recommending that people start 'small', as in lifting a small amount of weight at first. With a stoma, it is recommended that you start with small movements too: exercises that work just one part of the body, or one muscle group, rather than some of the bigger multi-joint exercises. So, that means strength moves that you can do seated and stationary, rather than ones where you're moving or getting up and down from the floor.

If you have a hernia already, or are concerned that you're at risk of one, avoid 'face down' exercises that require you to brace your belly muscles, such as a full plank and press ups and those where you have to brace and twist the torso.

Sarah Russell (honestly, you're going to need to read her book – it's so useful if you have an ostomy) prioritises what she calls a gentle core restoration programme first, before progressing onto more general strength training or further developing cardio-based activities.

There are some safe and specific strength exercises for those with an 'ostomy' in Chapter 4 (page 189).

'Ostomates'

Colostomy UK is a charity that you may already know – if not, have a look. They have completely embraced exercising for people with a stoma – who they refer to as their 'ostomates'. Their programme 'Active ostomates' has all sorts of resources and some online classes that are completely safe and suitable. They also tell the stories of their members who are swimming, running, and playing golf, football and even rugby with a stoma.[44]

Meet Renate

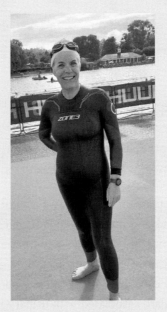

Figure 3 Renate wanted to get back to outdoor swimming

Renate was really active before her diagnosis of bowel cancer and particularly enjoyed open-water swimming. In the run up to her surgery she was convinced that she wouldn't be able to enjoy exercise once she had a stoma.

A few weeks after it was done, she came along to Maggie's and saw that there was a Nordic walking class. She decided to try it, but it took some courage to actually do it – she had a great fear of leaks while being out. 'It was a big step,' she told me afterwards. I remember walking with her that first time – tentatively, carefully. She was absolutely fine, other than that it poured with rain and we all got completely drenched. She continued though, and a little while later also tried doing a chair-based exercise class, using resistance bands for strength training.

She gradually built up the distance that she was walking and started joining '5k your way' to walk with us at parkrun. She somehow managed to stay active during weeks of indoor shielding during coronavirus.

She has since had her stoma reversed and has returned to her beloved swimming.

Pelvic floor training for men and women

One of the common consequences of cancer treatment, which doesn't get as much attention as it arguably should, is incontinence (and the fear of it).

It affects people much more often than we might realise, and surgery for bladder, prostate, colorectal and gynaecological cancers can cause it. It can be a consequence of brain or spinal cord cancers and of coughing associated with lung and oesophageal cancers. Radiation to the pelvic area can also irritate the bladder. Some chemotherapy drugs can cause stress to the bladder, and drugs that work on oestrogen-positive cancers are associated with urinary incontinence.[45]

In other aspects of life, incontinence can follow childbirth, and is experienced widely by both sexes as we age. It can really put people off exercising. If this is you, please don't be embarrassed. You're not alone.

Pelvic floor exercises

This is one aspect of exercise that we can absolutely take control over and is easily fitted into busy lives. You need no equipment, these exercises are quick to do, and nobody will know you're doing them. There is a section on how to train your pelvic floor muscles in Chapter 4 (page 132).

The exercises are a basis for training your pelvic floor muscles. As well as helping with leakage they are also an important – and often overlooked – aspect of strengthening the muscles in your core. They can help everyday moving and lifting to feel a little easier and can even contribute to a stronger, potentially less painful, back.

If you'd like some help in getting to grips with pelvic floor exercises, try the NHS Squeezy app – a phone app designed by specialist physios that takes you through the exercises and helps remind you to do them. It's really clever: www.squeezyapp.com.

If one of your concerns is around needing to find a toilet during exercise then I'd encourage you be completely assertive in checking that venues have one, and that they'll grant you access. Likewise, if there's somewhere on a route that you take regularly, such as a pub, my experience (and I've done it, many times) is that people are usually very accommodating, especially if they know your face already.

Macmillan have produced a 'Toilet card' – a discreet credit-card-size card with the request 'As a result of my cancer treatment I need urgent access to a toilet. Please can you help?'. It can be downloaded from their website.[46]

There are also several 'toilet finder' mobile phone apps that will check your GPS location and show you on a map your nearest public toilets.

Exercising after breast reconstruction surgery

Many women opt to have breast reconstruction, sometimes at the same time as the surgery to remove cancer, others a while afterwards. The procedures used are more complex than surgery without reconstruction, and as a result exercising afterwards needs to be done a little differently and with a little more caution. Most women are offered advice on what to do immediately after their surgery, and then advised to exercise gently, but not necessarily told how.

So, first things first. If you're reading this as someone that hasn't had the reconstruction yet, I would absolutely recommend some strength training as part of your prehab. Focus on strengthening the shoulders, chest muscles and abdomen. Do it right up until your surgery. The American website Breastcancer.org has some very useful information on what to expect immediately after surgery.[47]

Range of movement

Immediately after surgery, expect to be advised to avoid certain movements, usually around lifting, pulling and pushing. You will, however, be encouraged to perform exercises that gently help keep your arms and shoulders mobile. These exercises aren't shown in this book as they are specialised, and they differ patient-by-patient, surgeon-by-surgeon, and according to the specific procedure. So, I defer to your clinical team: either your surgeon, clinical nurse specialist or perhaps an oncology physio will talk you through the most appropriate exercises for you. Cancer Research UK have information on their website that shows some of the moves that are commonly used, according to the type of reconstruction.[48]

These exercises are really, really helpful in promoting healing and in avoiding frozen shoulder. Your movement is likely to be affected by the surgery for several weeks, perhaps longer, and so the exercises are crucial to maintaining as full a range of movement as possible. If you can, follow your clinical team's instruction to the letter. If you're unsure about any of the exercises, don't be afraid to contact the team, especially if there are specialist physios to advise: they want you to heal well.

If your surgery was some time ago, my recommendation is to return to these exercises first and go over them a few times to ensure that your muscles and joints have returned to full mobility.

As with exercising other parts of the body after treatment, we need to know first that the body has healed, secondly that it is flexible, and then we can start to work on strength.

Now I know that often fitness instructions will begin with a bland disclaimer to 'check with your doctor before starting'. Exercising after breast reconstruction is one situation where that's a really important step, so please do check that they think it's safe for you at this time. (They invariably are 100% supportive and will encourage you to go for it.)

First steps

Once we know you're okay to proceed, one excellent place to begin is with walking. As discussed in other parts of this book, walking can be soothing, it can be restorative, it's free to do and easy to just get on with. You can do it at your own pace – which ideally is fast enough that you're warm, and lightly out of breath, but still able to talk in sentences.

Do try to maintain good posture (both whilst walking, and otherwise). If you're able to stand tall, hold your shoulders back and your spine long, it'll encourage your abdominal muscles to work in supporting you. If your reconstruction involved the tummy area, walking with good posture could prove particularly helpful.

Getting stronger

In the first six to eight weeks, concentrate on your upper body mobility exercises. After this time, it is usually advised to be safe for you to return to 'normal activities', but you should avoid using resistance or lifting heavy weights.

Once you feel ready to, start to rebuild your strength. There are exercises specific to the different types of breast reconstruction later in this book (see Chapter 4, p. 165). Perform your mobility exercises first each time, as a warm-up, and then, using a very light resistance band at first, start building up. Ideally, do upper-body strength training two to three times a week on non-consecutive days. And do, absolutely start light and then build up slowly. It's fine also to exercise your abdominal muscles.

Stay aware – nothing should hurt and if it does, stop.

Exercising with peripheral neuropathy

Chemotherapy-induced peripheral neuropathy is a common problem occurring in approximately 30–40% of those treated with neurotoxic chemotherapy.[49] Affecting the hands and/or the feet, the severity can range from numbness to stabbing and/or burning pain. It can, unfortunately, last for months, even if treatment has finished. Not without reason, it can make exercising feel uncomfortable.

Peripheral neuropathy is also associated with a reduction in balance because the messaging system between the brain and the feet has been interrupted and this can render people more likely to fall.

In keeping with other aspects of 'exercise oncology', there is a growing body of evidence that exercise could have a rehabilitative effect with this condition. An initial study of women with breast cancer found it 'likely that an exercise intervention would be successful in attenuating symptoms of peripheral neuropathy and improving the overall quality of life (QOL) of breast cancer patients'.[50]

A later study led by the same team examined an 'exercise intervention' in more detail. Participants followed a 12-week programme in which they saw a personal trainer twice a week, doing 20–30 minutes of cardio training followed by a set full-body strength routine. The study found that, in those who took part in the intervention, 'overall QOL was significantly improved, and troublesome symptoms related to peripheral neuropathy significantly decreased'.[51]

Some other types of exercise that are recommended for people experiencing the condition are:[52]

- Stretching (to reduce inflammation) such as shoulder rolls, overarm reach, arm extensions.
- Walking. I know it might sound brutal to recommend walking to somebody with painful feet; however, if it is manageable, it should help increase blood circulation and muscle power to the feet and can help restore balance.
- Strength training, working major muscle groups (squats, lunges, hamstring curls).
- Balance exercises, such as heel-to-toe walking and slow knee raises, can help to decrease pain and improve coordination.

- Yoga – specifically somatic yoga, paired with meditation. A recent study reported that they 'may affect fear of falling and quality of life in cancer survivors with peripheral neuropathy'.[53]

Good kit can help

For strength training with peripheral neuropathy, I've found that wrist and ankle weights are really useful as you don't need to grip them with your hands or push against them with the soles of your feet. They are a good alternative to weights and resistance bands.

There are types of Nordic walking pole that don't have a wrist strap. They are designed specifically for people with discomfort to the hand, and that could be aggravated by the action of pressing the hand into the strap. I have found that people with peripheral neuropathy sometimes also experience very cold hands – poles that don't have a strap allow you to wear thick gloves.

There are strength routines, stretches and balance exercises in Chapter 4.

Chapter 2

When: the different phases of cancer

Exercising straight after diagnosis – 'prehab'

You would be forgiven for assuming that getting fit might be the furthest thing from a person's mind if they have just been diagnosed with cancer. It can be a time of absolute turmoil. If you are reading this as somebody who is going through diagnosis right now then, yes, it might not feel like going to the gym is top of your 'to-do' list. However, just as with many other aspects of exercise and cancer, there are significant reasons why it could be a really good idea.

Firstly, it can be an immense help in improving your sense of wellbeing during that 'in limbo' stage between diagnosis and the beginning of treatment. Exercise can help you keep your head together during difficult times. It can help distract you, help you sleep, help stimulate your appetite. It can really help how you *feel*. When I was going through my diagnosis, exercise was probably the most important factor in managing the gnawing anxiety I felt at the time.

So, why is it so helpful? There are several reasons. One thing that emerges from all the growing evidence and practice in this area is that, from a patient perspective, it can help you feel like you are taking back some control. Going through a cancer diagnosis is so often a time of great worry, and a time of waiting. Waiting for appointments, waiting for scans and biopsies, and of course, waiting for results.

And then waiting for treatment to start, which is often a period of several weeks. Patients may find themselves having to play a relatively passive role, waiting, and then listening, being told their results and their treatment options.

For many, it is terrifying. Waiting for treatment to start can feel like you are in No Man's Land. 'There's a myth that adopting a positive attitude can help. Well, it might, but you might want to rant and rave…, weep daily tears, or withdraw from the world.'[1]

The second significant argument for exercising straight after a diagnosis is that it can help your body to be able to tolerate whatever is about to come, and to recover more quickly from the treatment itself. If you are active in the run-up to treatment, you are likely to need to stay less time in hospital and are less likely to be readmitted.[2]

Encouragingly, you do not need months of preparation in order to feel the benefits. Macmillan Cancer Support say: 'The benefits of Prehabilitation can be seen in as little as two weeks. Prehabilitation empowers people with cancer to enhance their own physical and mental health and wellbeing and thereby supports them to live life as fully as they can.'[3]

Building the evidence base

The idea that people could, and perhaps even should, be physically active straight after a cancer diagnosis has been around for a little while but has gained significant traction recently, as the evidence base around exercise and cancer in general has grown and flourished.

Macmillan Cancer Support spearheaded this in the UK by bringing together an international body of experts to consider and develop guidance for what's become known as cancer 'prehab'. The Macmillan group have designed guidance on how it should be delivered and there are currently several trials underway across the UK. One such trial is across Greater Manchester, and the results so far have been startling.[4] It has received much praise and is being replicated now in other areas.

The Manchester project works like this:

- Patients are offered the prehab service within 48 hours of being diagnosed.
- The service has three distinct aspects: Exercise, nutritional advice, and support for mental and emotional health. It is strongly believed that all the three components are essential, and that they each contribute to the overall success of the programme.
- For the exercise part, participants do three exercise sessions each week which consist of high intensity interval training (HIIT) and strength training.
- Family and carers are encouraged to join in, partly so that they can then support the patient to be active outside the structured classes, and because they themselves are going through a difficult time and the programme may benefit them too.

When I was preparing for surgery, I based much of my approach to exercise on the work being done in Manchester. There is more information about what I did later in this book (page 78).

How to start your own prehab

I think it is important that any prehab plans are simple, structured and manageable. I would keep it simple because the period immediately after a diagnosis is one in which people are bombarded with information. There is often a great deal to do in preparation, around workplace arrangements, childcare arrangements, finances, etc. People can feel they need to get their 'house in order', anticipating a time when they might well feel too tired or unwell to do it.

So, my first recommendation is for a brisk daily walk, ideally outdoors. You might not feel like it every single day but try to make it something that you do as part of your regular routine. If you can, do this in a natural environment, because looking at trees and birds and seasonal change can really calm the mind. But it may well be that, in order to be practical, this is a part of a commute, or the school run.

If you can move faster than a walk, then go for it, or it might be that cycling's your thing. It just needs to be something to get you out of the front door, out of puff and warm. If you are not able to get outdoors, there are home-based routines later in this book.

Cancer treatment often results in people feeling that they are not as physically strong as they were beforehand. I see it a lot, especially in people's lower body strength. It can arise simply from having to sit or lie down much more than you are used to. People who have had surgery or radiotherapy around their upper body often report reduced strength in their arms and shoulders, and those having surgery or radiotherapy in the pelvic area often talk of reduced strength in their core. So, a useful part of prehab is strength training so that you begin treatment in the strongest position possible.

A little structure here is helpful, because strength training works best when it is performed well and with regularity. So, three times a week, on non-consecutive days (i.e., Monday, Wednesday, Friday) do something that challenges your muscles. This doesn't need to be time consuming or costly but getting as strong as you can could be really useful later on.

A note of caution – when prehab might need a rethink

For most people diagnosed with cancer, prehab is a great idea, but there are some situations that require a little caution. As with exercise during and after treatment, prehab activities need to be made extra safe for people with metastatic spread to the bones, simply to ensure that any risk of fracture is not increased. There are still all the potential benefits of exercise, of course, but just a few considerations:

- avoid activities where there is a greater risk of falling
- avoid contact sports
- avoid putting increased strain on the spine
- avoid excessive twisting and bending of the spine.

You can still train your back and core muscles, just with some caution. If you've been diagnosed with secondary cancer, please see the section about that later in this chapter (page 68), before you begin exercising.

Similarly, there are some considerations when embarking on a prehab programme if you have got reduced immunity. Just as Peter and I did below, avoid situations that could increase your risk of infection, such as public gyms, yoga studios and swimming pools.[5]

How Peter coped with watchful waiting

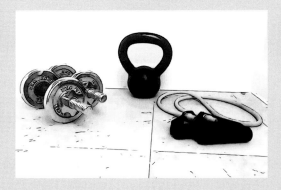

Figure 4 Peter needed to get stronger

Peter was diagnosed with T-cell prolymphocytic leukaemia (T-PLL) – an extremely rare and fast-moving leukaemia. Stem cell transplantation using bone marrow from a donor (preceded by gruelling drug therapy) is the only treatment option currently available. Although his leukaemia was aggressive, it was diagnosed early, and he did not have enough leukaemic cells in his blood (at the time of diagnosis) for treatment to start. So, he was put onto 'watchful waiting', a period after a definitive diagnosis and before treatment starts, in which you return to your cancer team regularly to monitor the disease's progress.

Also known as active surveillance, it is not easy to go through a period of repeated testing, in the knowledge that you will become increasingly ill and that only then will you have treatment. 'It is normal for watchful waiting patients to feel anxiety and a sense of helplessness.'[6]

Exercise is recommended for people on watchful waiting, for all the reasons outlined already. With Peter, we mixed interval running (short bursts, interspersed with walking breaks) and strength training. Prehab for leukaemia is still – as far as I could find – a relatively new concept. So that I could plan the best programme for him, I sought the advice of the international exercise oncology community through the power of Twitter. They told me to help him to build up his muscular power, so that his physical strength could help him tolerate the drug regimens and transplant that he would need later.

Peter's strength training was specific – small numbers (repetitions) of strength moves with the highest resistance he could manage. We used a heavy-duty resistance band outdoors, but in bad weather headed indoors and used weights in a gym. For Peter it was important to manage his increasing sense of tiredness as his illness progressed and he got nearer to treatment. We were also very mindful of his exposure to infection risk.

He underwent transplantation right in the throes of the Coronavirus pandemic. He's very tired, and I wouldn't want to understate the impact of his treatment on his strength. His steroid doses have been reduced, causing aches and stiffness too.

He is still exercising, gently for now, and has returned to work.

What else can you do to prepare for cancer treatment?

Personally, I took a leaf out of Manchester's book, and combined exercise with the best nutrition I could. Clinical teams, and support organisations like Macmillan and Maggie's, can help advise those who have inadvertently lost weight in the run up to diagnosis on how you can keep your strength up as much as possible by eating well. Exercise professionals can help with nutritional advice if you feel you would like to lose body fat ahead of treatment.

Also, if it is not stating the obvious, take care of your mental health. Again, there's support available from many sources, such as Macmillan Cancer Support, and organisations that focus on one specific type of cancer. Peter and his family found a great deal of support through specialist leukaemia organisations.

One of the things I see in many of the training sessions I do with people going through diagnosis and treatment, is that an outlet for emotions and stress is terribly important. Exercise can provide it and I often bring out the boxing gloves specifically to help people let off steam.

You might also seek out some calm, amidst the chaos. I have focused on physical activity that gets you out of puff and helps you to be physically stronger, because prehab evidence shows that it is effective. There is also a really important role for yoga, tai chi, Pilates – activities that can help you to relax and hopefully to feel calm. They can also help you to stay physically strong and balanced.

More than anything, let the time in the run up to treatment be for you. Self-care, as some may call it. Allow yourself time and energy, even if it is in small amounts, to wrench back a little control and devote some time to yourself. As someone once said, 'because you're worth it'.

During treatment – what's possible

Note: For this chapter, I am writing only about exercising during chemotherapy, radiotherapy and biological therapies. Exercising around the time of surgery requires specific planning, according to the site of surgery and the procedure involved, and needs to be too individualised for a book.

When I started out as a cancer PT, people – clinicians as well as patients – were still cautious about the idea of exercising during active treatment. The old adage of 'rest is best' had been thoroughly disproved for those who were post-treatment, and yet exercising in the middle of chemo or radiotherapy was often thought to be too much.

Fast forward almost a decade, and we are now seeing exercise bikes positioned in chemo suites, indeed a study examined the impact of moderate-level indoor cycling *during* chemo infusions. The basis of the study was that emerging, early evidence had indicated that if exercise is performed during chemotherapy infusion, patients might be able to absorb the drugs better, with less damage.[7] The study found that cycling whilst receiving a chemo infusion was both safe and feasible.

The above trial focused on moderate exercise, on the actual day of treatment. An earlier study looked at the feasibility and effect of high intensity interval training (HIIT), several times a week, for people receiving chemotherapy and found that a programme of high intensity cardiovascular and resistance training, plus relaxation, body awareness training and massage, led to reduced fatigue and improved vitality, aerobic capacity, muscular strength, physical and functional activity, and emotional wellbeing, but not quality of life.[8]

Many of the trials cited in this book were done with people with common cancers and I have found very little information about exercise for those with pancreatic cancer. One case study,[9] however, looked at training during chemotherapy for this cancer and concluded that 'regular aerobic and resistance exercise plus exercise during infusion can attenuate expected decline in physical and mental health with pancreatic cancer treatment and may reduce treatment side effects and have favourable effects on prognosis'.

There is some evidence around exercising during radiotherapy too: one study[10] described a home-based moderate intensity walking programme for men having radiotherapy for prostate cancer. The trial's control group – those not taking part in the exercise programme – found that they experienced a slight deterioration in physical functioning and a significant increase in fatigue by the end of their course of radiotherapy sessions. The men on the walking programme experienced the opposite: a significant improvement in their physical functioning with no significant increase in fatigue.

In 2020 a review of studies into exercise during radiotherapy[11] reported that 'Benefits related to exercise training have been shown in breast, prostate, rectal, lung, head and neck cancer patients undergoing radiotherapy. Therefore, exercise should be considered as a concurrent treatment alongside radiotherapy to alleviate treatment-related side effects and facilitate effective recovery'. The review recommended that training programmes should be tailored to the individual's medical condition, to their symptoms and to the specific side effects that they were experiencing.

An Australian study has looked at the habits of people receiving immunotherapy for advanced melanoma.[12] It reported that: 'patients are engaging in exercise while receiving immunotherapy, with the intent of mediating treatment-related fatigue.' This is interesting: for a long time one of the perceived barriers to exercising during treatment was that patients worried that physical exertion would make them more tired, not less.

So, we know it can be done safely, and we know that exercising when you're right in the throes of treatment, can bring benefits. But how to do it? And how should exercise be adapted for the periods when treatment is happening?

Exercising within treatment cycles

One aspect that many people need to work out is how they can adapt their exercise plans to fit into treatment cycles. They will often feel much less energetic, and more aware of the side effects of their treatment, in the few days immediately after each dose. This is true for most cancer patients for the duration of their chemo and other therapies. For those with secondary cancers, this is a long-term consideration. So, my advice would be to think of an exercise pattern that complements the treatment cycles, rather than one that tries to carry on despite them.

For example, some marathon training programmes run in three weekly cycles, where the runner would increase mileage in weeks 1 and 2 but then deliberately scale right back in week 3. This has been shown to help reduce the risk of injury and fatigue amongst long-distance athletes. They would follow that cycle for the duration of the training programme, which would normally be several months.

A cunning plan for somebody training whilst undergoing treatment could be the same: the few days immediately after treatment could be dedicated to active rest and recovery, some walking and good stretching; the middle week could be training at say 75% of the person's capacity; and the week immediately before treatment could be the most energetic. I'd plan to make their longest or hardest training session be a good couple of days or so before treatment, so that the body could rest before their trip to clinic.

Some other considerations

- As with many other scenarios described in this book, if you're embarking on an exercise programme during treatment, start gently and make the exercise light. Build up slowly but surely. Try keeping an activity diary to monitor your progress and energy levels.
- People are often advised to avoid swimming while having chemo and while having any treatment for leukaemia and other cancers of the blood. This is because treatment affects your immune system, and you may be more susceptible to any germs in the water.
- Similarly, you may need to avoid swimming during radiotherapy and shortly afterwards. Radiotherapy can cause skin changes which can be irritated by chlorine or chemicals in the pool.
- If you're having radiotherapy around the chest area, you may experience shortness of breath when you exercise. If this happens to you, do please check it out with your clinical team. Once they're comfortable that exercise is safe for you, have a look at the section on breathlessness in Chapter 1 (page 39).
- If you have experienced anaemia (low red blood cell count/haemoglobin) or neutropenia (low white blood cells) during your treatment, talk to your clinical team before beginning exercise – they may well encourage you to exercise but it's worth checking in to see if they have any specific recommendations for you personally.
- Likewise, talk to your clinical team if you're experiencing any ongoing pain, nausea/vomiting, diarrhoea, or any symptoms that cause you concern.

- It's fine to exercise if you're experiencing lymphoedema or peripheral neuropathy.
- Be gentle on yourself. If you're reading this but feeling like exercise is just too much for you now, then do please cut yourself some slack. Have a read of the section on active rest and recovery in Chapter 3 as a starting point (page 124).
- If you can, do what you love. Cancer treatment is hard enough, without you also having to do exercise that you don't enjoy.

Exercising with a Hickman or PICC line or Portacath

Understandably, many patients with a Hickman or PICC line or PortaCath are hesitant, yet it is fine to exercise, and to work on maintaining your physical strength, if you have either of these inserted. You're advised to avoid any heavy lifting – the guidance is to lift no more than 5 kg/10 lb. The trick, as ever, is to work out a safe level to start, and then begin by using only light weights or a light resistance band, and then gradually and steadily build up.

You are advised not to swim with a PICC; you can with a port. You should avoid contact sports with both.

With a PICC, especially if it's inserted in the lower arm, you should avoid exercises that require the elbow to bend sharply (e.g., bicep curls) and beware of large, forceful movements, such as a golf swing.

Otherwise, with either a PICC or port, its fine to move your shoulder and chest muscles, and to do exercises to strengthen those areas. Whenever I am going to begin to train somebody with one, we first check that it feels secure to them, before exercising. Then we'll do some small gentle movements (reaching upwards, pushing outwards, raising the arms out to the side etc) to see whether they feel the PICC/port move as they go through an increasingly full range of movements. (People rarely feel anything that concerns them, but I find that doing this helps reassure us both that we're safe to proceed. If anyone says that something doesn't feel right, we avoid that type of movement.)

There are some strength exercises that form the start of safe strength training with a PICC/port, see Chapter 4 (page 158).

Biological therapy – exercising through trastuzumab (Herceptin)

Women who have been treated with trastuzumab (brand name, Herceptin) will know that it can have an impact on the heart, and because of this they have regular heart scans during treatment. Beyond the scans, your clinical team can advise you on the safety of exercising.

Women I have trained while they're on Herceptin sometimes say that they feel like their breathing is a little laboured, as if they were trying to walk against a strong wind, although this often affects them when they're resting rather than when they're moving. Normally I find that they are advised that it is safe to exercise while they're on Herceptin, but with caution. I have trained women who have steadily built up their ability to walk, then walk briskly, then jog in intervals, whilst taking the drug. But do start gently and work up very gradually.

Meet Odile

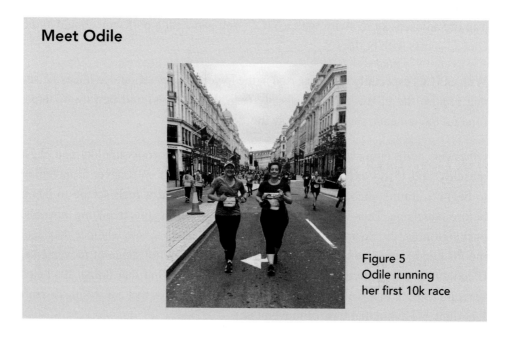

Figure 5
Odile running
her first 10k race

Odile worked her way through a 'Couch to 5k' programme during her treatment of chemo then surgery and Herceptin. She also Nordic walked, used a skipping rope, did strength training and used a weighted hula hoop to help with core and back strength and flexibility. She had a PortaCath – and so when we first started training we assessed which arm and shoulder movements felt comfortable for her and we based her upper body training on those she felt happy with. She listened to her body and, particularly on the days immediately after each infusion, she dialled back her exercise a little, and then built up during the rest of the three-week cycle. Sometimes she repeated one of the weeks in her Couch to 5k programme and then progressed to the next week when she felt ready.

She is doing brilliantly and just completed her first 10k race since her diagnosis. After her port was removed, we started boxing.

When exercise is not advised

If you are currently having cancer treatment, guidance,[13] advises no exercise in the following circumstances:

- On the actual days you have intravenous chemotherapy, or within 24 hours, and none prior to blood draw (I'm sorry, I know this is inconsistent with the study about cycling during infusions. The guidelines pre-date the study).
- If you have very low blood counts.
- If you have a fever of 38 degrees C or above, or if you have an acute infection. Wait till you have been symptom-free for two days.
- If you experience severe nausea, vomiting or diarrhoea.
- If you have chest pain, shortness of breath, dizziness, lightheaded disorientation or blurred vision.
- Or if you have other conditions than could preclude exercise, such as angina, heart failure, diabetes and others that are currently unstable.

While living with secondary cancer

It is well known, and well documented, that exercise can be really helpful for anyone who has had a diagnosis of cancer, indeed Macmillan Cancer Support says 'physical activity can benefit patients at all stages of the cancer care pathway'.[14]

My observation is that so much of that focus and knowledge is on those who only had primary cancer. The many people living with secondary cancer are very often overlooked, in terms of information and of support so that they can safely and effectively be active.

Again, there's evidence to support the value of physical activity in all people with secondaries. Wilk *et al.*[15] conducted a literature review around the advice and range of interventions available for people with metastatic cancers. They concluded that exercise could really help improve outcomes, but that advice and exercise plans should be tailored to the needs of the individual. They recommended that: 'Physical activity should become a standard component of every metastatic cancer care plan.'

Fatigue, and muscular strength

One very commonly experienced side effect across many types of secondary cancer is fatigue, and this is often accompanied, and exacerbated, by reduced functional, muscular strength: if you have lost weight during treatment then there's every chance that some of that weight was muscle. This can impact greatly on your sense of strength – daily activities just feel so much more difficult if the muscles that carry you are not as big and strong as they once were.

As well as helping some things to feel easier, strength training can be helpful in restoring energy. Many people wouldn't necessarily see the link but having more muscle on your frame has been shown to help reduce cancer-related fatigue. A study cited by Macmillan in their advice for people with secondaries 'compared a resistance training programme to passive physical therapy in 60 patients with spinal bone metastases, showed that resistance training was able to improve functional capacity, reduce fatigue and thereby enhance quality of life over a six-month period'.[16]

I believe that we should all think of strength training as an essential part of our lives, and for the rest of our lives.

Exercising within treatment cycles

One aspect that many people need to work out is how they can adapt their exercise plans to fit into treatment cycle, which, for those with secondary cancers, is a long-term consideration. So, my advice would be to think of an exercise pattern that complements the treatment cycle, rather than one that tries to carry on despite it. There's more detail on this earlier in this chapter (p. 63).

Make good quality rest and recovery a part of daily life

Often overlooked, restorative and active rest periods are hugely important in the long term and are a completely valid component of any plan for a more active life. This isn't simply loafing about on the sofa (although of course that does have its place). Active rest can be walking, stretching, gentle movements that encourage the body to repair. I would recommend developing good practice around rest and recovery to everyone, and especially to anybody hoping to be more fit and active while living with secondary cancer. It will prove its value to you.

Don't over-train

For those who've been regularly active in the past, there can be a huge adjustment to make. It can be terribly difficult to accept limitations that weren't there before your diagnosis. You might find yourself yearning for how your body felt, and how it could perform, before cancer appeared in your life.

It can be tempting to over-train. You may well get a sense of instant satisfaction – that sweat, the endorphin high, the sense of your body really moving, or working hard. Going back to what you used to do, before all this...

Some people, improbably, can still exercise extremely hard during cancer treatment, but my experience is that it might come with a high price and lead to the injury bench. Deciding the degree to which you are willing to limit the intensity of your exercise is a highly personal choice – and it is indeed *your* choice.

Two fabulous women and a hashtag

Jo Taylor, founder of After Breast Cancer Diagnosis, is living with advanced breast cancer. As well as managing an especially useful website and blog, Jo runs residential exercise retreats for people affected by breast cancer, and she is a tenacious advocate for improved treatment for people with secondaries. She teaches Nordic walking and is currently training women with breast cancer to become Nordic walk leaders. Jo recommends you have an exercise buddy, and that you do what you love. I couldn't agree more. You can find Jo at www.abcdiagnosis.co.uk.

Deborah James, aka Bowel Babe, broadcasts as part of the 'You, me and the Big C' team. She is living with advanced bowel cancer. She, rather fabulously, ran a 10k race in her bra and knickers, to encourage body positivity. The link here is to a great film where she talks about what exercise has meant for her since her diagnosis, including a bit about the impact on her lung tumours: www.youtube.com/watch?v=-jtffYNC-rE.

#busylivingwithmets: Twitter and Instagram have some real gems, and this is one. I like it because it's mostly used by regular folks who are, as it says, recording their everyday lives. Expect to see plenty of realistic updates, from people who are busily, actively living with secondary cancer.

Please see the section on active daily living in Chapter 3 (p. 91) – moving little and often as a way of life as opposed to exercising as a separate entity. Active daily living (ADL) involves choices and lifestyle changes that help us to move more as part of our everyday activities.

Adapting exercise for people with secondary spread to the bones

Our main concern when there is secondary spread to the bones is around reducing the risk of fracture, and so recommend activities that are low impact and non-contact, and with attention on reducing any risk of falling. Weight-bearing exercise (i.e., on your feet, transferring your weight from one foot to another) is useful as it can help to minimise bone density loss.

If you experience any increase in bone pain, report it to your clinical team.

It is important to protect the spine, so avoid sharply twisting or bending/arching your back. One question I've been asked is how to strengthen the back and tummy muscles whilst avoiding such twisting and bending. The trick is to focus on exercises that require the back and torso to remain stable as opposed to exercises that demand movement e.g., bringing the knees towards the chest rather than bending the chest towards the knees.

There are some exercises to try in Chapter 4 (p. 188).

Adapting exercise for people with spread to the brain

Some people with a spread to the brain are advised by their oncologist to avoid inverted movements (handstands, headstands, downward dog in yoga) and beware of positions that can cause dizziness.

Otherwise, it's sensible to mitigate against the risk of falling that could be prompted by dizziness. This doesn't need to be anything too complex, just make sure you've something stable to grab if you need it. As a trainer I'm advised to be aware of a risk of injury for anybody experiencing seizures – my experience is that anyone in this situation is normally highly aware themselves, but it's something to bear in mind, especially if you're increasing your activity levels or trying new activities.

A stationary bike can be helpful and they're more versatile than many would expect. You can use them for a gentle pedal (watching the TV if you get bored) and they can be useful during active rest periods. Sessions on an indoor bike don't have to be sedate though – try a spin class. There are loads of online options now. Some are free, others such as Peloton can open up a whole new world of activity. I often do this one: www.youtube.com/watch?v=lFbjsRvjF-A . (I take no responsibility either for the background music or for the distinct lack of diversity of body shapes by the way.)

Many people find their balance is affected by cancer treatment and this can be especially the case for people with brain cancer or with spread to the brain. Exercises to improve your balance and coordination can be reassuring. They work best if you do them often. There is a balance routine in Chapter 4 (p. 190–194).

Adapting exercise for people with spread to the liver

Many people are reported to encounter considerable fatigue with liver secondaries, and often nausea or loss of appetite (or both). Active daily living may be the most helpful plan during any periods of particularly difficult fatigue. I'd advise anyone feeling nauseous to stop exercising, until the feeling has passed. Talk to your clinical team if it persists or if you're eating less than normal.

Adapting exercise for people with spread to the lungs

Many people with secondary cancer in the lungs experience breathlessness, and this can make exercising seem impossible, or at least uncomfortable. I know that many clinical teams offer advice on breathing techniques, and exercises to help. The section on breathlessness in Chapter 1 (p. 39) might help you to feel in control of your breathing during exercise.

Paying attention to having good posture can be useful for all of us, and particularly those with lung cancer or lung secondaries. My observation is that people who've had cancer treatment involving the lungs (and breast) often develop a rather protective way of holding their posture, as if they're trying to shield the area.

One form of exercise that I would highly recommend to anyone with lung cancer, or with secondary spread to their lungs, is Nordic walking. It is gentle, yet effective cardiovascular exercise, and many people say that having the poles can make walking feel more manageable. Part of the reason for this is that the poles help you to stand up straight. Nordic walking is also a lovely way to enjoy outdoor and sociable exercise – good for the soul.

Seated cardio

I think chair-based exercise is often underrated. It is useful if your mobility is affected either by cancer or by life in general. It is a way of moving without the risk of falling, so it can be helpful for people with reduced balance and with peripheral neuropathy. If you have secondary cancer in your bones, the chair can help stabilise your spine and hips.

Seated exercise sessions are often focused on the gentler side of exercise and that, for many, can be lovely, and can be enough. Have a look at the classes run by your local cancer support centre. Since the beginning of the coronavirus pandemic, online seated classes have popped up in many places – I run one on behalf of Maggie's, using Zoom.

Seated cardio exercise can be surprisingly hard work and it's possible to get out of puff, and feel your heart rate going up, even though you're in a chair. You can increase the intensity of the exercise by wearing weights attached to your wrists and ankles (helpful for neuropathy in the hands) or hold light dumbbells as you move – see the seated routines in Chapter 4 (p. 133).

After (primary) treatment – when the circus leaves town

This is the point at which this book started and for many people it's a time that is surprisingly challenging. Our expectation beforehand may be that it's a time of jubilant celebration: it may well be, but in reality it often is more complicated than that.

It can feel like an anti-climax after months of intense activity and it can feel worrisome to suddenly find you're on your own after being in other people's care. There can be a palpable feeling of abandonment. My first boss at Maggie's, Bernie, described it as 'when the circus leaves town', when everything goes quiet. This is a time when many people's emotions wobble as they have time to reflect upon what just happened.

There is evidence to support these observations. A study by the Mental Health Foundation[17] described an emotional 'false summit' at the end of cancer treatment. It found that mental health problems often arise at the very end of treatment, rather than earlier, at a time when there can be less support available to help.

Dr Frances Goodheart talks about how we no longer allow time for 'convalescence',[18] and just expect to get straight back into the swing of things without giving ourselves the chance to recuperate. End of treatment is a time of adjustment, often before going back to work, yet some of the side effects of treatment – fatigue, reduced strength, peripheral neuropathy, for example – will still be felt, and for a few months.

In the context of exercise, my advice would be to follow the ethos throughout this book: start gently, keep it manageable, integrate being active into your emerging routine. You may very well still be experiencing side effects, but your body (and mind) are not having to endure the impact of more treatment and so recovery will come. Allow yourself some time and space to convalesce.

Clare's story

Shortly after treatment for colon cancer, Clare – aged in her 30s – suffered cardiac arrest that was caused by chemo drugs. She was advised to start exercising but, like many others, needed to find ways to start carefully, and to work progressively.

A few weeks into our time training together, I asked Clare if she would like to try something new, and she was open to giving it a go. It turned out that this gentle, thoughtful, emerging writer, was a demon with boxing gloves!

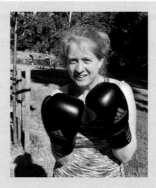

Figure 6
Clare boxing

This is one of my very best examples showing that we should do what we love.

Towards the end of life

Exercise for people who are in the terminal stage of their cancer is important and yet, alas, often overlooked. As with all the other aspects of the disease, staying active can help to support our sense of wellbeing towards the end of our lives. Most of the content of this book applies completely to those whose cancer has advanced and has been deemed 'incurable'; this can be a period that (hopefully, of course) lasts for many years during which time the cancer may be in remission or dormant. Beyond that, though, and specifically, how could we define the most helpful approach to exercising once cancer has become terminal?

For guidance here, I have looked to the World Health Organization, and the UK National Council for Palliative Care, whose shared 'Principles of Palliative Care'[19] can, I believe, be applied to physical activity. They include:

- Providing relief from pain and other distressing symptoms. Gentle movement that dynamically stretches our muscles and elevates our heart rate can help to offset pain and muscle tightness. It can also help to prevent reduced strength through muscle loss, encourage better sleep and improve appetite.

- Affirming life. Staying active may help us to continue to do what we love, and to continue to enjoy experiences that create memories both for us, and for those around us. We can use movement for its instant mood-enhancing feel-good quality.
- Offering a support system to help patients live as actively as possible until death. Increasingly there are activities within hospices and cancer care centres, such as walks, mediation and mindfulness sessions, and exercise and yoga classes, that have been specifically developed for people with terminal illness. Many hospices have gyms, some have swimming pools.
- Aiming to enhance quality of life.

What's best?

In terms of what type of exercise is best, I hark back to 'doing what you love'. It makes sense to spend precious time and energy on activities that we actually enjoy. Beyond that there is limited guidance specifically on how we best would exercise at this stage. Advice from the Australian Cancer Exercise Toolkit cites a study that found the benefits of exercise in advanced cancer did not appear to depend upon the mode of exercise (e.g., aerobic vs strength). As a trainer, they advise me to devise training programmes based on the client's goals and preferences.[20]

We know that exercise can help us cope emotionally. Several organisations recommend, and provide, group exercise, and they can be really valuable for the peer support that comes with it. I see this regularly with the classes I run at Maggie's. Marie Curie quote one of the attendees at their hospice gym classes:[21] 'Everyone is in the same boat, all trying to get your limbs to work, and that's what I really, really like about it. I live alone and it gets you out and it gets you meeting people.'

Regardless of the stage we're at, people with cancer will often find that exercising helps them to gain a sense of control when in a situation in which they can feel powerless. This is as true here as it is from day one, at diagnosis. Karen Turner, a physiotherapist at the Marie Curie Hospice in North London, conducted her own research within the hospice gym to understand whether people's participation in exercise programmes had affected their quality of life. They reported that they 'felt that by coming to the gym they were able to reclaim some control, giving them renewed confidence and hope for the future'.[21]

One issue that does arise is the preservation of strength and balance. Falls are particularly pertinent towards the end of life and, if possible, prevention is key. An evidence review found that 50% of patients diagnosed with advanced cancer fall during the subsequent six-month time frame. The review reported the benefits of specific fall-prevention exercises to include improved health status, functional mobility, or muscle strength.[22]

Roger's story

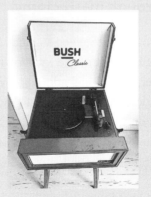

Figure 7
Roger and I
used jazz

Roger was my most senior client so far – we trained together until he died, in his mid-90s. When we met, he was living with advanced prostate cancer and dementia. We used music and dance – something he'd loved as a younger man, which helped him to reminisce and remember good times.

His exercise programme was adapted as his strength and energy levels changed. Initially we went Nordic walking in a nearby park (the poles helped him to feel more stable on his feet). We'd stop midway and have a good chat and do some 'sit-to-stand' and shoulder rolls on a park bench.

After a couple of nasty falls, we moved our sessions indoors and developed a routine that incorporated gentle stretching and strength, and balance using his dining table, kitchen worktops and doorways as support. In time he started to use a walking frame in between exercise 'stations' (we travelled from room to room in his house, doing a different exercise by each doorway) but importantly, he kept moving, and dancing.

He suffered a stroke, and from then on, he used a wheelchair but still we exercised – gentle chair-based marching, stretching and using light resistance bands. And as ever, having a good old chat.

My story – moving through mastectomy

The Coronavirus pandemic of 2020 changed so much for so many and will continue to do so for a long time. At the start of the lockdown, I was working full time as a cancer rehab fitness trainer, a job I had adored for more than seven years. I was fit, and mostly worked outdoors. As the realities of lockdown and social distancing became clear, I knew I wouldn't be working much, but I imagined I'd use the time to update my website, do the bookkeeping, finish that book (this one!) I had been writing for several of the aforementioned years.

And then, three weeks into lockdown, I found a breast lump. Quite by accident, after I had been doing a load of boxing, holding weights, with a couple of clients online. I thought I had just inflamed one of my pectoral muscles.

I was wrong.

For me, going through a cancer diagnosis felt odd, almost dreamlike. A bit of a blur now, although at the time each waking minute was experienced acutely. Doing it at a time of global crisis just made the whole thing even more surreal.

Keeping my head together

I learnt for myself the value of cancer prehab, especially its incredible ability to help you to keep your head from exploding. My exercise of choice is to run. I am not fast, but I find a 5- or 6-mile plod, somewhere as pretty as I can get to, just sorts me out.

I experienced profound anxiety as I was going through the diagnostic process, especially during the time when I needed to make decisions about my treatment. During the hours and days immediately after my diagnosis I was thrown right off kilter. I guess it was shock. I tried a little run but just could not muster the energy.

The following day I was so anxious that my breathing was fast and shallow. I couldn't handle coffee as it made me completely jittery, and I had to resort to deep, mindful breathing just to regain my composure. I gardened, which always soothes my soul.

I started to keep a diary of my emotions and I also noted my activity levels, and it was extraordinary: on the days that I exercised in the morning I was less anxious for the rest of the day. That's endorphins for you. I opted for shorter runs, normally 3 or 4 miles, on most days.

Looking after my (physical) strength

I was lucky, as I was already physically strong, but I knew that my surgery would impact upon the strength in my arms and shoulders, so I worked on exercises that would allow me to go into surgery with strong muscles in the areas that I thought would be affected.

My programme of upper body exercises is illustrated in Chapter 4 (p. 151).

Strength to function

I had been given a leaflet of physiotherapy exercises to do after my surgery. I already knew how helpful they could be. I have worked with people who swear by their effectiveness. I have also worked with women who have suffered months, even years, of pain, frozen shoulder and a limited range of movement as a result of their breast surgery. So, while I was in hospital waiting for my surgery, I practised them, so I knew what they were meant to look and feel like.

Extra self-care

Many years before we knew what we now do about cancer prehab, a wonderful cancer surgeon called Professor George Hanna taught me something. He would counsel all of his patients to 'train' for their surgery day as if it was what he called their own personal Olympics. He would encourage them to do everything in their power to go into surgery in the best shape possible. He was way ahead of his time.

So, for my Olympics I made my diet as good as I could. Loads of fruit and veg (after surgery I upped my protein intake, particularly red meat too). I ate as little sugar as possible and made sure I was well hydrated. My plan was not complex, and if felt good to be looking after myself. Similar to exercising, it was something that I could take control of, at a time when other things were totally out of my control. I reduced my alcohol intake to almost none.

Straight after surgery

This might sound extreme, but I walked home from hospital after surgery. I'm lucky – my home is less than a mile from my hospital bed and it felt rather good, to get some fresh air on the day I was discharged.

I walked almost every day after surgery, although the first couple of days were just tentative short walks near to home. Walking with chest drains was fine but I must admit I felt vulnerable. This is unusual for me. I normally feel pretty invincible and certainly not fearful of people, but the combination of surgical wounds, drains, and Covid meant that I was very edgy and feared being bumped into. That passed once the drains were out.

I did my physio exercises religiously, and they helped. My ability to move my arm came back fully – it did take a few weeks, mind. Here is a little film of the exercises

I did at first: https://youtu.be/jmDNpV2UP5s. Once the drains were out, I could use larger movements without fear of moving the muscles around my ribs too much.

Along with my physio exercises I also did some gentle back and neck stretches, as I was stiff from having to sleep differently. I was surprised by the degree to which I felt my chest muscles when I moved and stretched. I really had not realised how fundamental they are to our movement.

I was soon able to increase the range of movement in my upper body exercises. I built on the exercises that the physio had shown me and added in small versions of the movements from my pre-surgery strength programme, but without any weights or resistance. This film shows the exercises I did: https://youtu.be/qlMIrEgDc44.

5k my way

I have been a part of '5k Your Way, Move Against Cancer' for a while, and I set up the lovely group that canter around Southwark parkrun once a month.

On day 4 after my mastectomy I got a bee in my bonnet, as you do, and I decided that I was going to aim for 5 km on foot every day during my recovery. It is a nice round number, and a distance that I know well and understand. It's an hour's brisk walk (for me) and just over half an hour's run.

And so that is what I did. Just walking at first, and then with Nordic walking poles. The poles felt marvellous, and along with all the evidence about their effectiveness for women who've had breast cancer surgery, I can also say from experience that they helped me progress my range of movement through the shoulder and also I think they helped to make the puffiness from surgery go down. (Poles when used properly are known to help encourage lymphatic drainage.) The poles helped me to increase the intensity of my daily exercise session.

Now, don't get me wrong – this was not all plain sailing. There were some days when I felt really down. Sometimes my arm felt uncomfortable as I exercised (there was a dragging sensation as if my limb might come away from the shoulder joint). And the numbness from surgery felt really odd, like my sleeve was twisted around my arm, even though it wasn't. A mastectomy wound feels as if you're wearing an exceptionally uncomfortable bra.

On Day 13 I overdid it. Walked too far, used the poles too enthusiastically, didn't have my then obligatory afternoon nap. I had no idea that 'just' surgery can leave you so very, very tired. So, I took a rest day, only doing my physio exercises, and then went for a gentler walk without the poles the day after that.

And then, on day 21, my daily 5k included a gentle little jog – just a few paces at a time, really tentatively. (I was trying to work out how to run without letting my chest bob up and down. It must have looked hilarious). The following day I did my first proper run, and it felt epic. I took the photo below after that run.

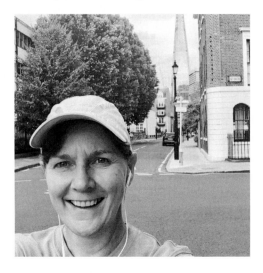

Figure 8 My first run after surgery

Weights – where many fear to tread

After breast cancer surgery many women don't know how they can safely rebuild their upper body strength without causing injury and without triggering lymphoedema. The general rule is that you can return to 'normal activities' six weeks after surgery and can start to increase resistance (i.e., the amount you lift) after eight weeks.

I started using light hand weights during week 6 and have gradually built up since then. I made a film of these exercises: https://youtu.be/TruXQPaCvXo.

What next?

I guess we might be divided into people who want to go back to 'normal' after treatment for primary cancer, and those for whom it is a catalyst for change, for a better quality of life, or to do those things they'd always wanted. I'm not sure yet which path I'll take.

I have been able, cautiously, to go back to practising yoga, although I opt for the gentler stuff these days. I definitely have less energy than I did before my diagnosis and subsequent menopause. The drug I'm on (tamoxifen) makes me a bit stiff and achy, but I can live with that.

I am deeply grateful for the care I have had, and the kindness and support that came my way.

And I feel well.

Chapter 3

What to do, and how

How to start – walk a mile a day

So, we know the reasons to do it, we know that being active is generally A Good Thing, and that for everybody with a cancer diagnosis, it's a particularly good idea. We also know that almost without exception, and despite any caution or trepidation you might be feeling, the chances are that you *will* feel better once you've done it.

I think that the best first step in trying to get active after a cancer diagnosis is simply that: take a first step by going walking. It's what I did.

Aim to leave the house and walk as briskly as you can for a little while, take a rest midway then walk back. Many people would walk a mile in 20 minutes or so, and it can be a manageable and quite a neat goal to walk a mile every day – briskly, mind; no dawdling.

I've trained many people who'd find this a breeze, and others for whom a mile a day would be a significant challenge. (See also the section on chair-based exercise in Chapter 4 – p. 133. Your 'mile' could be measured in time rather than distance and could well be performed in a chair.)

Marie's story

When I first met Marie, she'd recently finished chemo after breast surgery. The treatment had left her exceptionally tired, and she found that it was all that she could do to walk to the post box at the end of her street. She began to walk every day, and, wisely, recruited a neighbour to walk with her. They didn't go far at first, but they went out, reliably, every day. Their walks built up gradually in length, and it proved to be a lovely opportunity for them to seal their friendship. The daily walk offered a sense of routine after a period of complete upheaval.

After a while, Marie came along to a Nordic walking class at the Maggie's Centre. At first, she took it very gently, and would have a rest on a bench along the towpath as her buddies went ahead a little and then came back to pick her up. Marie stuck at it and bought herself a pair of walking poles so she could go Nordic walking on other days as well as with the group. Over the weeks and months she became steadily fitter. She would be at the front of the pack, chatting, and wouldn't be completely pooped by the end of the walk.

This is her crossing the finishing line as she completed her first 5km Race for Life.

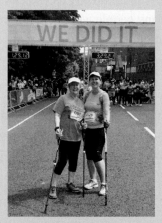

Figure 9 Marie finishing her 5km Race for Life

So, here's the plan: a good, brisk, purposeful walk, every day. A full 20 minutes of active walking, more if you can. This can be a remarkably simple thing to do, but it can have a profound effect.

It might be that it's part of a regular commute (imagine how wonderful it would be if we could all walk to work). I stress that the walk needs to be brisk – try to walk at a pace that feels as fast as you can comfortably manage.

You should become a little warmer as you walk. Feel your breathing change so it becomes a bit deeper – but stay comfortable enough that you can still speak in sentences.

How hard should you be working?

Cancer can leave a legacy of tiredness.[1] It varies from person to person, of course, but most people find they have low energy. Many also experience muscle loss, and just generally feel that they're not as strong as they were. As described in the section on fatigue in Chapter 1 (p. 15), there's some evidence to show that exercise at a 'moderate', level of exertion, (with your heart rate about 70% of its maximum) would be a good level to aim for.[2]

This may, of course, feel like waaaay too much exertion for you, especially in the earlier days of getting fitter. If that's the case, don't worry; just make sure that you continue to push yourself (gently) and go as quickly as you can, as if you were in a bit of a hurry. Aim for consistency first – so you're doing something most days. This will help to build your stamina, and strength, so you will in time be able to do more.

Is it safe to start?

Normally, if I'm meeting a new client, I have to ask them to fill in a little form just to confirm that it's safe to proceed. It's a common practice across the fitness industry and you might have completed something similar if you have joined a gym or been to one as a visitor. The questions I ask are standard:

- Do you have a diagnosed heart condition?
- Has a doctor ever recommended only medically supervised exercise?
- Do you ever experience chest pains during or after exercise?
- Have you suffered from chest pains in the last month?
- Have you ever lost consciousness or fallen over as a result of dizziness?
- Do you have a bone or joint problem that could be worsened by exercise?
- Do you currently have any sports related injury?
- Do you, or have you ever, taken medication to control your blood pressure or to treat a heart condition?

Sometimes the form feels quite inappropriate as we will invariably have already had a long chat about the client's health history but still, it is sensible to ask. If you, now, would answer 'yes' to any of the above questions, then I recommend that you check with your GP or one of your clinical team that it's okay for you to exercise now. It normally is absolutely fine, but it might be that they recommend some form of caution or adaptation as you start.

Mindfully as you go

If you're going to be exercising outdoors, try to get into the habit of looking around as you go. Soaking up nature and the beauty around you can do wonders for your state of mind. If you're walking every day you will see things progress as the seasons change – buds become blossom, leaves change colour. Whatever changes are going on, try to notice them, even if you feel you're walking somewhere that's not particularly special. Some of my Nordic walkers recently spent 20 minutes or so, in November, in central London, mindfully spotting all the flowers and seeds they could see as we walked. It was a lovely, enriching experience and there were, of course, all sorts of treasures to find that we'd have otherwise overlooked.

We know that mindfulness can have a significant effect on our immediate mood and on our long-term mental and emotional wellbeing. Making your daily mile mindful could reap more benefit than you might expect: one study found that 'mindful walking in nature may be an effective way to maintain mindfulness practice and further improve psychological functioning'.[3] So, more bang for your buck.

Enlist a walking buddy: Borrow My Doggy

Some people love to walk alone – it offers solitude and a time for a bit of reflection, to let your mind wander. As a keen runner, I particularly love to go for a long steady run along the Thames path, on my own. It gives me a bit of mental space to mull things over, or to watch the birds, look at the tide, watch things pass me by.

Some people, however, find it doubly hard to motivate themselves to exercise if they're on their own and so a cunning plan is to have a training buddy, like Marie did. They'll help you to commit to a time to go out, and you'll egg each other on.

I think 'BorrowMyDoggy' (www.borrowmydoggy.com) is a marvellous idea for those of us who'd love a dog but can't have one full time. BorrowMyDoggy is an online membership scheme that matches dog lovers who have a bit of spare time with nearby dog owners who have a hairy friend available for extra walks.[4] It sounds like a win-win situation to me, and scientists would approve: a study looked at activity levels of those who had a dog and compared them with those who did not. Guess which group walked the most, and walked more briskly?[5]

Meet Rita

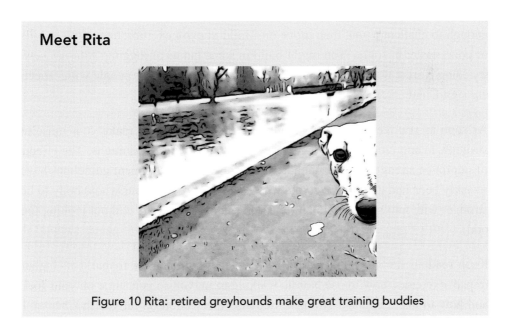

Figure 10 Rita: retired greyhounds make great training buddies

Rita, the retired greyhound, belongs to one of my clients who is exercising after breast cancer and with a form of multiple sclerosis. Greyhounds make excellent training buddies as, contrary to popular belief, they are docile and really rather lazy (apart from when they spot a squirrel). Having a dog means that your motivation to exercise outdoors is non-negotiable: you have got to go out, probably twice a day, regardless of the weather.

Rita's owner recently told me: 'by far the most impactful thing for my walking rehab has been Rita. Not only does she get me out, but my balance has improved enormously due to her erratic pace, changes of direction and sudden stops right in front of me.'

Too tame for you?

It might be that the idea of walking daily feels a bit too tame for you, especially if you were regularly active before your cancer diagnosis. That's fair enough. My best advice is to try it, especially if it's still early days during or after treatment. Make this your foundation to build on, and once a brisk 20-minute walk doesn't feel like enough to challenge you, then move on. Build in extra exertion by adding in hills or going faster in spurts. You might build in some bursts of jogging. Alternatively, try using Nordic walking poles as their benefits, especially for people with cancer, are significant.

As soon as you feel ready, start doing exercises that help to make your muscles stronger. I can't emphasise enough how important strength training is. The effects of improved strength are substantial, so much so that government guidelines have recently been updated to reflect the benefits.[6] You can train your whole body to be stronger with minimal equipment (and you can do it outdoors without looking too odd).

Keep reading for information on how to start running, how to build in higher impact exercises, how to use Nordic walking to maximise your time on your feet, and how to make yourself stronger. See also the section on fatigue in Chapter 1

(p. 15), which looks at how to exercise when you're tired, and the section on active rest and recovery later in this chapter (p. 124), which has ideas on how to keep your pecker up on low-energy days.

Active daily living and exercise 'snacks'

When we think about physical activity, we often focus on specific sports or types of exercise, overlooking other activities that involve movement and that can help bring about all the benefits of 'exercise' without necessarily wearing Lycra or going to a gym.

Active daily living (ADL) involves choices and lifestyle changes that help us to move more, to sit still less, and to sit less still. The idea is that we move little and often, like getting off the bus a stop earlier than you need to. It can be helpful for those short of time as you can work out ways to fit it into your day.

ADL can be helpful in managing cancer-related fatigue. It can be effective – you teach your body to use energy and improve its strength as a way of life rather than in deliberate chunks of time. It becomes 'how you do things' rather than a separate, deliberate facet of your daily routine. You can be really creative with this approach and develop your own personal plan of attack.

It is an excellent plan for those who don't enjoy exercise per se, and it can feel less overwhelming than the idea of starting a full exercise programme. It would make an excellent place to begin to exercise during treatment. In time, ADL could provide gains in strength and energy which might support you in increasing the intensity of your exercise, should you wish to.

ADL can in some ways be about us making life less convenient for ourselves; indeed, in the days before we had the technology we have now, we had far less need to even consider making like more active. Remember having to get up out of your armchair to change a TV channel?

Other examples of ADL are:

- parking in the furthest space, rather than the nearest
- taking the stairs rather than the lift, or climbing whilst on an escalator
- getting involved in active neighbourhood projects such as communal gardening
- using a standing desk, rather than sitting down to work.

Minutes spent moving prompted by the methods above all count towards your 150 minutes a week (see section on 'exercise prescription' opposite).

Exercise 'snacks'

Another way to increase your levels of activity in small amounts is to start doing 'exercise snacks' – quite literally something small and light rather than a big feast! Exercise snacks are intended to be very brief – perhaps 20 to 60 seconds long – and to be done as frequently as you want to. Also sometimes referred to as 'movement breaks', the idea is being studied by some of the scientists involved in devising high intensity interval training (HIIT)[7] who found that physical activity in short fast bursts can be surprisingly effective (see the HIIT section later in this chapter – p. 113).

So, rather than ADL which is intended to become part of how you naturally do things, exercise snacks are deliberate. Some examples of exercise snacks are:

- Practise controlling core muscles or do pelvic floor exercises between stops if you're standing on public transport.
- Sit with good posture and try to hold it for a given period of time – see if you can eat an entire meal whilst sitting up straight.
- Sit on a Swiss ball. Stand on a Bosu.
- Do squats while you're washing the dishes, lunges while cleaning your teeth, stretches while you wait for the kettle to boil.
- Move during the advert breaks when you're watching TV.
- Take a break while you're working to climb the stairs or walk briskly to the end of the garden.

Cindy is Rita's owner and she's brilliant at exercise snacks. As well as walking the dog two or three times a day, she has started to use a skipping rope and is trying to jump higher. She does 10 jumps whenever she goes to her hallway to put her shoes on. She also sits on the floor to put her trainers on in the morning, and practises getting back up again. I think this is genius and a huge confidence booster for anyone afraid of falling (and not being able to get up).

The exercise prescription – how much, how often?

I hope, through this book, to convince you that we all can be physically active, and purposefully keeping our bodies strong, for the rest of our lives. But how do we break this down into manageable chunks, and turn such ambitions into everyday reality? How can we know how much will be 'enough'?

Guidelines for prescription

Guidelines for all people with cancer in the UK are based on recommendations from the American College of Sports Medicine (ACSM), which state that we should all aim for:[8]

- at least 150 minutes of aerobic exercise (i.e., getting out of puff) per week
- at least two sessions per week of resistance (strength) training on non-consecutive days
- stretching our major muscle groups every day when possible.

The guidelines go on to recommend that exercise programmes should be modified around each individual's health status and the degree to which they're affected by side effects. At a minimum, people with cancer are urged to 'avoid inactivity' and to be as physically active as possible.

Some people, on hearing the recommended '150 minutes' worry how on earth they'd fit that into their busy lives. The secret is to break it up – it's half an hour a day, five days a week, with exercise snacks if you need to do it in small chunks.

Rate of perceived exertion (RPE)

After the prescription of how much, we also need to consider how hard, how intense, should the exercise feel. To gauge the intensity of aerobic/cardiovascular exercise, there are several scales that we can use to self-score, to measure how hard we're working. The one I prefer to use is arguably the simplest. Rate how hard you're working on a scale of 1 to 10 using Table 2.

Table 2: Rating how hard you are working

Rating	1	2–3	4–6	7–8	9	10
Described as	Very light	Light	Moderate	Vigorous	Very hard	Maximum effort
Feels like	Anything beyond sitting/ lying still	Movement that you could maintain for hours, with normal breathing	Exercise that you could maintain for a considerable time. Breathing heavier, but you can talk in full sentences	On the verge of uncomfortable. You're short of breath but could still speak in short sentences	Not able to do this for long. Can barely speak, breathing very heavily	Flat out. You could only work at this level very briefly. Can't speak

Most recommendations for aerobic or cardiovascular exercise, and many of the clinical studies described in this book, are based on moderate exercise. One of the reasons that I like this scale is that it is subjective – it's about how you feel, at the time and compared to how you normally feel rather than comparing yourself with other people. Broadly though, most Nordic walkers report that they're working at a moderate level. When I'm running with a client they'll usually say they're between 7 and 9.

Training your muscles to become stronger

In terms of strength training, one of the reasons why it's so important to learn good technique is that ultimately what you're trying to do is exhaust your muscles. They then need to rest, and during that time of rest they repair, and rebuild to gradually become a little stronger. We need to make sure that we do this safely, to avoid injury.

When we move our muscles against resistance, our brain will eventually get a message that the muscle is tiring; the brain will reply 'enough!' and we stop. It's the point at which the weight feels too heavy, or you know you need to stop for a moment.

Whether we're using our bodyweight, resistance bands or weights, the art of strength training is to select enough resistance but not too much. Unless it's stated otherwise, throughout this book you're looking for the right amount of resistance so that your muscles are tired after 10–12 repetitions. You might then rest from that specific exercise for a few minutes and then do the same number of repetitions.

Training programmes will typically contain a range of exercises that work your lower body, upper body and/or trunk. Large 'compound' movements that require several joints to work simultaneously are often recommended as they are more time efficient than ones that only work one part of you or one muscle group.

Design your own training plan

You may well want to simply exercise and take part in activities when you fancy them, or when the opportunity arises. If you want to really focus it helps to have some sort of goals, or intentions, and often a plan is a helpful way to map out how to reach them. Table 3 is an example of a personal training programme that I might design for someone starting out.

Table 3: A personal training programme

	Type	Activity
Monday	Cardio, strength and full body stretch	45-minute Nordic walk. RPE 5–6 1 set of 8–12 repetitions of the following: Squat, lunge, wall press, glute bridge, chest press, shoulder press, standing ab curl, seated knee raise. Have a rest in between exercises if you need to Stretch afterwards
Tuesday	Rest	Yoga, any physio or rehab exercises, or gentle stretching
Wednesday	Cardio, strength and full body stretch	Zoom-based group class Stretch afterwards
Thursday	Rest	Yoga, any physio or rehab exercises, or gentle stretching
Friday	Cardio, strength and full body stretch	30-minute walk. RPE 4–5 1 set of 8–12 repetitions of the following: Squat, lunge, wall press, glute bridge, chest press, shoulder press, standing ab curl, seated knee raise Stretch afterwards
Saturday	Cardio and stretch	Up to 5 km walk or jog. RPE 6–7 Stretch afterwards
Sunday	Rest	Yoga, any physio or rehab exercises, or gentle stretching

If it would help you, please take this example and adapt it to your lifestyle, time constraints and preferences. A programme is best set for a period of eight to 12 weeks, but review it as you go, and reassess your progress before developing it further.

Once you feel that you can progress to make it more challenging, a training manual issued to professionals by CanRehab recommends that you:

- Develop strength training by first increasing the number of repetitions of each exercise. So, using the exercises listed in the plan, you might try doing each of the exercises in turn and then repeat the whole lot, or build up until you can do 15–20 of each in one go.
- Don't skimp on your recovery time in between exercises or between strength sessions. The rest time is important.
- When you're ready, start to increase the amount of resistance very gradually. This can be achieved by, for example, holding a hand weight while you do squats and lunges, holding a resistance band over your hips as you do the bridge, shortening the resistance band for the arm and shoulder exercises, or raising both knees at once, rather than alternating them.

(The exercises are illustrated in Chapter 4.)

How to progress your exercise

As personal trainers we are given the acronym FITT to consider as we help our clients to progress; this stands for:

Frequency – how often the client is training
Intensity – how hard, how fast, how heavy etc
Time – how long they're doing it for
Type – the type of exercise and the variety.

We are advised to normally increase only one component at once, so that we can assess the impact of that change. I would urge you to do the same. Training programmes work best when they are truly progressive, and that progress is gradual and measured.

Be your own personal trainer

Design your own programme using Table 4 – select the type, duration and intensity of your cardio sessions. Choose a range of strength exercises from those described throughout this book, paying attention to any particular considerations for you personally, such as the side effects described in Chapter 1. Think about how and when you'll rest, how this can fit into treatment cycles if you're having them, and use the full body stretch in Chapter 4 (p. 195). Happy planning!

Table 4: Design your own training programme

	Type	Activity
Monday		
Tuesday		
Wednesday		
Thursday		
Friday		
Saturday		
Sunday		

For the reluctant, the self-conscious and the tired – barriers and how to overcome them

You might be surprised to read that, just occasionally, I don't fancy exercising. Sometimes I do not want to get cold/hot/wet/sweaty etc. and sometimes I simply cannot be bothered; I'm too tired and want to lounge around.

There are some classic barriers to exercise that are very commonly experienced, and that are totally understandable for someone who has had a cancer diagnosis. Alongside tiredness I often find that people are afraid that they will do the wrong thing and might injure themselves or exacerbate side effects. Some examples of this are around wounds after surgery, stomas and ostomies, people experiencing peripheral neuropathy, people with secondary spread (especially to the bones) and those whose heart or breathing is impacted by their cancer treatment. It is more than reasonable to be cautious. This book will hopefully support anyone experiencing any of those side effects to feel confident that they can be more active, and that they can choose what they do and enjoy it.

Self-confidence tricks

Some people are very, very self-conscious about the prospect of exercising anywhere, and perhaps even more so about doing it outdoors or in a public place. They are embarrassed or think they will be judged by other people and this feeling can be exacerbated by cancer treatment as it can disrupt our body confidence and self-image.

That's understandable. Now, I don't want to sound glib – it would be easy to say 'well other people don't matter'. (They don't, though.) But here is one observation. I stand around in parks and open spaces with clients all the time and typically they are doing an exercise while I look on, encourage them, hold the stopwatch etc. I often notice the reactions of passers-by and always they are positive. It's often a respectful nod or smile. Sometimes people will offer a couple of words of encouragement or say 'Good on you' or 'I need to do that' as they pass.

Put yourself in charge

One of the reasons people will choose to work with me as a cancer exercise specialist is that they know I understand that cancer treatment can limit what they are able to do. Some folks have reported feeling 'bullied' by trainers to work harder and to constantly be making improvements, setting goals, or progressing to do more difficult things. I've noticed this often with my younger clients – sometimes they will have been expected to keep up with their peers even when that's simply too much to ask. I think this happens mostly when there aren't too many visible signs of cancer treatment to remind others of their history.

Now, I would not want to limit anyone's expectations, and throughout this book I talk about progressing, and developing strength and fitness. I do, however, think it's important to accept that cancer treatment does have a huge, varied and often long-lasting effect. Our intentions to be stronger and more active shouldn't become something that feels overwhelming or impossible.

So, if you can, please aim for a sense of self-efficacy around your approach to exercise. It can be whatever you choose it to be. Your aims can be broad – to simply feel a bit better – or to become more active more regularly, rather than to walk or run a particular distance or lift a certain weight. If you're exercising during treatment, your intention could be around *maintaining* strength and levels of activity rather than increasing them.

Time: there aren't enough hours in the day

A lack of time is a very commonly held reason why we don't fit in as much exercise as we intend to. Finding time when you are also tired can be doubly difficult. For those that struggle with time, I would suggest looking for opportunities that are either time-efficient, or convenient. If you can use a journey you regularly do and convert it into your exercise – the work commute, or after the school run, it might be easier to fit it in and make it a habit. If there aren't decent facilities to shower and change at work, then walk or run home: it also acts as a de-stressor, a gentle come down, ahead of the rest of your day or evening.

Types of exercise that are time efficient are often ones that involve quick bursts of activity, such as a HIIT session, or using a spinning bike. For the reluctant and self-conscious, you can do HIIT in your living room, or garden – it doesn't need to be in a gym-based group.

Using a skipping rope is also a wonderful option for the time strapped and it is something you can do little and often and build up. Skipping is excellent cardio exercise, and the jumping is excellent for preserving bone density (provided it's okay for you to do high impact activities). If you use social media, @kathyjumps is someone I follow. She started skipping to regain her confidence after giving birth. Whenever her babies slept, she would skip. She is now impressively fit and posts imaginative, fun, realistic films of her routines, with coaching notes. Check her out on Instagram.

It can also help if you purposefully 'book' your exercise time with yourself, to help develop an internal sense of commitment. Lizzy Davis, a lovely fellow cancer exercise specialist, coined the phrase 'Schedule it in rather than squeeze it in'. It's valuable, and it's worth allocating our time to do it.

Do it with a buddy

If you want to start, or go back to, exercising, then getting some support can be really helpful, especially if you don't know how to start or if you're struggling to find enough motivation to keep going. If you can enlist a friend or family member as your exercise buddy, you will spur each other on.

Or join a group – such as those operated by Maggie's Centres, many hospices and Macmillan Move More. There's some evidence to show that you're more likely to stick to your intentions if you exercise with other people rather than alone, and you'll get the added bonus of social support from kindred spirits. One clinical study found that: 'Group exercise classes offer a less intimidating approach to fitness. Not only can it be a place where participants learn helpful ways to increase their daily activity, but they also have the opportunity of fellowship with other patients who are in a similar stage of treatment.'[9]

Men with prostate cancer may find it particularly encouraging to exercise in a group setting. One review of exercise programmes specifically for prostate cancer patients found that they tended to prefer to exercise with their peers, in supervised, structured programmes.[10]

Advice from my cancer rehab exercise class

I asked the lovely crowd at one of my online sessions for their advice to anyone with cancer who was just embarking on exercise and their comments are shown in Figure 11.

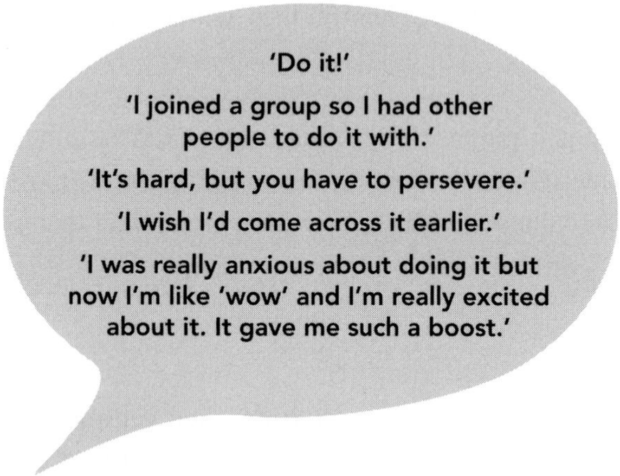

> 'Do it!'
>
> 'I joined a group so I had other people to do it with.'
>
> 'It's hard, but you have to persevere.'
>
> 'I wish I'd come across it earlier.'
>
> 'I was really anxious about doing it but now I'm like 'wow' and I'm really excited about it. It gave me such a boost.'

Figure 11 Advice for people starting exercise

See also the section on 'Do what you love' later in this chapter (page 105). I can't stress enough how life-affirming it can feel to be active in a way that you enjoy.

What to do if you are having a 'down day' or are struggling to get going

There are some tricks I have learned in order to convince myself (and others) to 'just do it':

- Put on your kit. Even if you don't go and exercise straight away, it should help prompt you.

- Allow yourself to just do a little bit. If a whole workout, or session, feels too much, it is fine to change your plans and opt for something that feels less overwhelming. Sometimes I tell myself I will go for a run but will intend to keep it short. Invariably once I get going, I do the full distance anyway.
- Make it feel like a treat – a bit of 'me time'. Go somewhere different, or beautiful, for your exercise rather than the usual route. I sometimes run one way along the river Thames, then catch a boat home marvelling, like a tourist, as we pass under Tower Bridge.
- Have something indulgent or nourishing waiting for you at the end: a soothing bubble bath or particularly good cuppa. I find that a really good, gooey chocolate brownie works well.
- Sometimes, you might simply need a day off, and this is absolutely fine. Perhaps have a good stretch or do a little yoga, but do please cut yourself some slack if you need to. I hope that exercise becomes a habit for life and, in order for that to be practical and sustainable, sometimes you do need to rest and put your feet up. I often run better, and much more strongly, if I have had a couple of rest days. There's more about this in the section on 'Active rest and recovery' later in this chapter (page 124).

When not to exercise, what to avoid and when to be cautious

We know, categorically, that exercise after a cancer diagnosis is a good idea on so many levels. It is more than a decade since the American College of Sports Medicine (ACSM) concluded that 'cancer survivors could safely engage in enough exercise training to improve physical fitness and restore physical functioning, enhance quality of life, and mitigate cancer-related fatigue'.[11] However, the ACSM produce guidelines for exercise professionals like me that are used globally, and they have some specific cautions to note when people who have had cancer treatment are planning to exercise – see Table 5.

Table 5: ACSM guidelines

Issue	Specific advice
Bone loss/bone metastases	Avoid movements that involve excessive bending or twisting. Opt for low impact activities and be mindful to avoid the risk of falls. New or worsening bone pain should be referred to your clinical team.
Lymphoedema	Wearing a compression garment has traditionally been recommended. ACSM now advise that it is up to individual preference.
Older adults	Some physical problems that can result from treatment – such as muscle weakness, sarcopenia, and fatigue – may be accelerated in older adults. Before starting exercise, have a fitness and functional assessment with a physio or specialist trainer to find the best level to start at.
Ostomy	Empty ostomy bag before exercising. Strength training should be low resistance and under supervision to ensure good lifting technique and good posture. Do exercises that help protect against hernia. Avoid isometric exercises where you have to 'hold', like the plank. Ensure against dehydration. Wear a shield if doing contact sports.
Peripheral neuropathy	Be mindful of the risk of falling – use treadmills with a handrail. Stationary bikes and water-based exercise are good if your feet are affected. Wrist weights can be helpful if grip in hands is affected. Do balance training.
Stem cell transplant	Recovery at home is recommended. Avoid gyms until full immunity is restored. Opt for low intensity, short but frequent sessions and progress gently.
Clusters of symptoms and side effects	During cancer treatment, and for those with advanced cancer, be mindful of multiple side effects (e.g., fatigue plus pain plus poor sleep) and report to your clinical team if they worsen.
Sun safety	When exercising outdoors, practise good sun safety.

Do what you love

Of course, some people just do not enjoy exercise. For many the idea of going to a gym is anathema. Fair enough. Instead, I'd recommend looking for other ways for your body to move – dancing, gardening, active daily living. There may well be some activity that you've done in the past and that you'd like to return to, or something that you've harboured an ambition to do one day. It doesn't have to be a big thing; whatever you would like, for you, and for your body. Whatever you want to put your time and energy into. Figure 12 shows all the activities that my clients have returned to, or worked towards, after a cancer diagnosis.

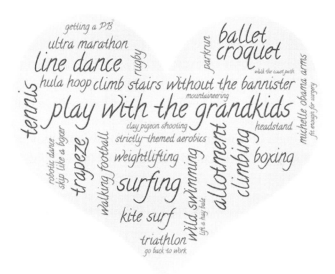

Figure 12 Some of the goals we've used

Alternatively, find something new and learn, through coaching if need be, to do it well, as that can help build confidence and a sense of satisfaction at the same time as helping you to feel fitter and stronger. I have, for example, taught boxing to many people (one was a lady aged 84), who simply didn't have the opportunity when they were younger. It is highly satisfying, and a great workout.

There are some people who have a lifelong dislike of exercise, stemming from their experiences in school sports, or through other enforced exercise. The trick here, I find, is to make it enjoyable, and often, therefore, non-competitive. It is one of the reasons that parkrun appeals to so many – anyone can do it, everyone is welcome, and the only person you're competing against is yourself, if you want to.

I remember once training with a client who was just coming to the end of her time in the British Army. Over a period of time she learned to love running, against her own expectations. Beforehand, at school and in the army, running had always been under duress, but she found that if she didn't pressurise herself in the pursuit of speed, and if she allowed herself walk breaks, she actually enjoyed it.

The joy of Zumba

Zumba is a dance-based form of exercise, devised by a Colombian dancer and choreographer in the 1990s. It has become a global fitness phenomenon and you can find classes everywhere from YouTube to your local village hall.

It is a fabulous weight-bearing, fat-burning cardio way of moving and is really good for anyone who isn't particularly fond of running/walking-based activities or cycling.

However, the main thing about Zumba is that it is fun. The music is mood-boosting, it's absorbing as you have to really concentrate to learn the choreography, and it is rewarding when you grasp the moves and fall into rhythm with your instructor and classmates.

Unlike some other exercise forms, Zumba classes don't tend to be stuffy – they're friendly and inclusive, and it doesn't matter if you go wrong. In fact, Zumba can help to restore coordination and balance and you'll find yourself moving in multiple directions and faster than you might have thought possible.

I highly recommend it for anyone who's looking for something that's uplifting and hard work, yet suitable and adaptable for more or less any of us.

Meet Deedee

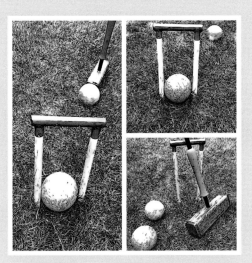

Figure 13 Deedee used a mallet and hoops to get her oomph back

Another of my clients is nicknamed after, to use the sporting phrase, the GOAT, in her chosen field ('Greatest Of All Time'). Deedee is exercising after thyroid and breast cancer. She discovered a love for croquet, and has become an accomplished, and I might say highly competitive, club and league player. Although croquet is a gentle sport, it requires a great deal of control (and, therefore, upper body strength), so her training programme is geared around strength and fitness to help her play at her best. Croquet is also outdoors, sociable, weight-bearing – it ticks lots of boxes.

And that, my friends, I believe is the key to lifelong fitness: finding an activity that you love to do.

Nordic walking – perfect exercise

I use Nordic walking as an integral part of the training that I do – at some point almost everyone I train does it. The reason I'm such an advocate is that Nordic walking is brilliant exercise in general, and near perfect for people with cancer. It worked for me during my recovery, acting as a stepping stone from gentle walking to running again. I'm convinced that it helped reduce the post-surgery swelling and helped get my arm moving fully again.

Based on cross-country skiing, Nordic walking is an outdoor activity that will work your whole body without impacting too much on your back, knees and ankles. This is exercising at a level at which you can chat, have a giggle, and at the same time become stronger and get a real sense of satisfaction.

Nordic walking works the whole body. What's more it's hard enough, but not too hard – it can be adapted to suit everyone's individual fitness levels. For most people it will feel like a very spirited, energetic walk, but without that 'I can't breathe' feeling that sometimes happens with running.

What's special about Nordic walking?

The difference between Nordic walking and walking briskly, or with trekking poles, lies in the way we use the poles to propel the body forwards. Trekking poles, also called hiking poles, are used to support people's balance while they walk, whereas Nordic poles are used to assist momentum. Nordic poles hit the floor by your feet, and you push them down and backwards; they therefore cause your body to move up and forwards. You wear a special strap that attaches to the pole, so there's no need to grip it hard, and you can't drop it.

You strengthen your shoulders, arms and core with this movement, and it's this propulsion that gives you the added oomph to walk faster and stronger. You then get into a fabulous cycle where the poles help you do more, and you use your body strength to push them, thus building your strength and fitness and therefore meaning you can do more and more.

And, *and*, it feels nice. I've known people say it makes them smile, or that they feel like they're flying. It makes walking feel good.

Why, specifically, in relation to cancer?

Nordic walking is an accessible and low-cost way to exercise, and as such it can simply be a way of starting to live a more active life.

It is, however, a clever sport: the amount of exertion involved in Nordic walking can be particularly helpful in overcoming fatigue and I find that many people can Nordic-walk at the ideal, 'moderate' 70% HRM. Not only this, but I find that Nordic walkers can sustain 70%, or thereabouts, for longer than they would without the help of the poles. It also helps to restore good posture, to burn fat and to build, or re-build, muscles.

We know how important weight-bearing exercise is to bone health after cancer treatment, to help prevent osteoporosis. Nordic walking is weight-bearing, so it ticks that box. Most advice about weight-bearing exercise focuses on the spine, pelvis and femur (thigh bone). Over the years I have wondered whether the action of striking the ground with the poles would improve bone density in the arms. A recent study suggested that it certainly could.[12]

Of course, an inevitable benefit of Nordic walking is that it gets us outdoors and therefore can offer a huge boost in mood. You get a sense of the seasons, hear birds singing and top up your vitamin D levels. Nordic walking is often done in groups (better at first if you're self-conscious about using the poles) and these tend to be highly sociable.

Many cancer support organisations, like Maggie's, offer Nordic walking as part of their programmes of activity. Something that's struck me over the years that I've run classes for Maggie's and Breast Cancer Haven is the calibre of conversations my walkers have with each other. Nordic walks can offer a rare chance to chew the fat with people who've been in the same boat as you, and know how you feel, without you necessarily needing to explain.

Women with breast cancer

There is a growing body of scientific evidence around Nordic walking as a rehab tool, and lots specifically around women recovering from breast surgery. The use of poles helps target the muscles that are often affected by breast surgery and the rhythmic action of the arms and shoulders can encourage and support lymphatic drainage. A recent study in Italy said: 'In order to choose a physical exercise having complete efficacy against breast cancer treatment effects on the side of treatment, particular attention should be paid to Nordic walking. Nordic walking has been reported to achieve balanced postural changes in breast cancer-related treatment postural disorders, increases in upper extremity strength, improvements in cardio-metabolic and respiratory measures and has been used in the prevention and treatment of upper limb lymphoedema.'[13]

The benefits relating to upper body lymphoedema are impressive. A study carried out in the Netherlands showed that after 10 weeks: 'patients' vitality had improved, whereas perceived shoulder symptom severity and limitations in daily activities had decreased… data indicated that range of motion of the affected shoulder improved significantly within 10 weeks of training. Group interviews at 6 months' follow-up confirmed that patients had appreciated the physical and psychosocial benefits of the intervention.'[14]

And anecdotally, my clients with upper body lymphoedema who take up Nordic walking tend to find that their symptoms improve, especially if they manage to learn good technique. I swear it helps keep my lymphoedema swelling to a minimum.

So how to start?

As with other types of exercise, you'll get much more out of it if you do it well. This is particularly true for women wanting to increase their shoulder mobility or manage lymphoedema. It's important to learn how to swing your arms from your shoulder – like a soldier marching – rather than bending the elbows.

There is a detailed step-by-step guide to Nordic walking in Chapter 4 (p. 146).

If you'd like some help in getting started, most instructors offer free trial sessions for people to give it a go, and they run technique classes so that you can finesse your technique. Look online at nordicwalking.co.uk or britishnordicwalking.org. uk for your local instructor in the UK or, if you're in the London area, contact me. For readers in Ireland you can go to https://nordicwalking.ie and/or https:// nordicfitnessireland.com.

Happy Nordic walking. I hope you can enjoy it as much as I do.

Upper body strength – a gentle start

As a personal trainer I get asked about this a lot. If you've had a period of inactivity during cancer treatment, then you may well feel that your arms and shoulders aren't as strong as they used to be, regardless of which areas of your body have been affected by treatment.

As outlined earlier, all types of cancer treatment can leave you feeling fatigued, and in many cases weakened. One client told me that chemo made her muscles feel soft, like putty. Some people are concerned about how their arms and shoulders look, but more often I find that they're discovering that lifting, reaching, sometimes just holding something heavy, has become more difficult.

How soon can you start?

If you've had surgery, I would advise you to err on the side of caution and wait until eight weeks afterwards (unless your surgeon/nurse says otherwise) just to be absolutely certain that the wounds are fully healed deep down, as well as on the surface of the skin. At the time of surgery you may well be given mobility exercises – in the case of the upper body around keeping the shoulders mobile – and they can be performed immediately after surgery. I did mine while I was still in my hospital gown – I was very keen to keep as much movement in my shoulder as I could.

Once you've reached eight weeks or more after surgery, I recommend using resistance bands (rather than weights) and your own body weight, and to build up a basic routine that, in time, can be expanded. Try to do this three times a week, on non-consecutive days so that your muscles can repair on the days in between – it's the combination of rest and resistance that causes us to build stronger muscles.

Start with resistance bands

There are exercises to improve upper body strength using a resistance band in Chapter 4 (p. 151–158). It is the routine that I used for my post-mastectomy strength training. When you're using a resistance band, let the slack, non-used part of the band just fall away, rather than wrapping it around your fingers as this could affect your circulation.

Once you're familiar with how to do each exercise, adjust the length of the band so that there's enough resistance that doing 10–12 repetitions of each exercise is enough. Make it shorter in order to work harder, lengthen it if an exercise feels too difficult. What you're aiming to do is to tire the muscles each time.

None of this should hurt though, and if you're feeling a twinge, perhaps through cording or frozen shoulder, then ease off and discuss it with your specialist nurse or physiotherapist.

Some cautions

These exercises are chosen specifically to help with problems with shoulder mobility and are safe for you to do if you're at risk, or suffering, from lymphoedema (just make sure that you follow the usual precautions).

It is fine to do strength exercises during and after radiotherapy – but be mindful of any skin discomfort. Stop if any of these movements cause you any pain and check in with one of your clinical team if you're concerned.

It's also safe to do some upper body strength moves if you have a Hickman or PICC line or Portacath, and these are described in more detail in Chapter 2 in the section 'During treatment – what's possible' (p. 65).

The mantra: start light, do it well, build up gradually

The best way to train to increase your strength is to start small and then gradually build up over a period of time, perhaps two or three months, so that you are challenging yourself steadily. As the weeks pass you should find that your strength increases, and you may well need a stronger band.

Be a perfectionist about your technique – do these exercises really well and stop if you find that muscle tiredness (the slight burn you can feel from lactic acid) is making you perform them incorrectly.

HIIT – what's it all about then?

HITT (high intensity interval training) has become an extremely popular way to exercise, principally because it can be highly effective, but it's also time-efficient – fabulous for those pushed for time or wanting to see quick results. Although interval training (interspersing bouts of activity with short, regular rest breaks) has been around for a long time, HIIT came into sharper focus over the last 15 years or so, after scientific studies found it to be, potentially, a way to become much fitter through doing short exercise sessions. One seminal study found value in participants exercising for only 2–3 minutes at a time, so you potentially could get fit in just a few minutes a week.

Studies have variously shown that HIIT can significantly increase both aerobic and anaerobic fitness and can significantly lower insulin resistance. It can help to make the muscles stronger and to burn fat.[15]

For a long time, and certainly while I was training to work in cancer rehabilitation, it was thought that HIIT would be too much for people with cancer. It was thought that working at such high levels of intensity could cause fatigue, which would have been completely counterproductive. Plus, although there is a growing body of clinical evidence to support the benefits of HIIT, most of the original studies were carried out on healthy, young (often male) participants and they would exercise to a point of significant discomfort during the trial sessions. There's an argument for a little caution in understanding how this otherwise convincing evidence applies, in real life, to people with cancer.

However, a study published in 2019,[16] reviewing the current evidence around the effects of HIIT for people with cancer, found benefit: that doing HIIT could be as helpful as more moderate types of exercise, and was better than no exercise at all. The review also found that people who used HIIT during and after cancer treatment were more likely to burn fat than those doing more moderate exercise. The review concluded that: 'HIIT might be a time-efficient intervention for cancer patients across all stages of therapy and aftercare.'

So, it's another tool to add to the box, if it's something you think you might enjoy.

Isn't that what that journalist was doing when he had a stroke?

Yes, it is – in 2013, Andrew Marr suffered a stroke after an extremely hard interval workout on a rowing machine. This sounds alarming, of course, but there were other factors involved – he'd had two 'mini-strokes' before, and reportedly was under a lot of stress in his life when it happened. In response to his experience the *Nursing Times* gave some great advice on what could be learnt from Mr Marr's experience, which centred around understanding the link between high blood pressure, stress and TIA (mini-stroke): 'We do know that high blood pressure itself is the single biggest cause of stroke. Until more research is done on specific triggers, we'd suggest getting your blood pressure checked and taking steps to keep it under control – exercise can help with that.'[17]

So, if you're reading this and if you've had a history of high blood pressure (or TIA), or are very unfit, then a gentler start to getting fitter would be safer and may feel less overwhelming. If you think this applies to you, please have a good chat with your GP, oncologist, or a specialist trainer to make sure that you opt for types of exercise that will be both effective and safe, for you, for now.

What do I need?

HIIT isn't a specific exercise or type of move, but instead it's a method of how you balance exercise intensity with periods of rest. The studies described were based on bodyweight cardio exercises, but interval training works really well with walking, running, cycling, swimming etc – any activity where you can easily alter your working intensity. The weight-bearing cardio routine in Chapter 4 (p. 138) can be performed as a HIIT session. This is an example of using the FITT approach to progressing exercise that was described earlier.

You need to be able to keep a close eye on a stopwatch without having to stop and fiddle about with it. There are lots of free apps to download onto a smartphone that will beep at given intervals and these are really helpful.

Do please be a little cautious if you have cancer in your bones or unstable blood pressure, and make sure that you've had sufficient healing time from surgery – as described earlier in this chapter. For example, if you're being protective of your bones, stick with the low impact exercises, just with increased intensity.

What intervals to use?

I'd recommend this as a starting point: warm up properly first – this is really important if you're going to use high intensity bursts of activity.

Then go through the whole routine on p. 138–145, doing each move as energetically as you can for 40 seconds, resting only for 20 seconds to get your breath back. Use your 20 second break to get into position for the next exercise – move briskly and steadily through the whole routine without stopping, if you can.

You should feel like you're working at a high RPE (rated perceived exertion) – it should feel manageable, of course, but ideally aim for an effort rate of 8 or 9 out of 10. Make sure you do the exercise properly though – don't compromise your posture or technique.

Take plenty of time to cool down and stretch afterwards.

Running: you can, honest

Running has never been more popular than it is at present. Many marathons (and increasingly shorter races) have had to introduce a ballot system in order to fairly allocate the available places. Parkrun, which started in 2004 as a bunch of mates timing each other's runs in Bushy Park, has grown into a worldwide phenomenon. There are now over 3 million parkrunners.[18]

Many people, however, find the idea of running completely daunting. For some it's the challenge of keeping going if you're running alone, for others it's the thought of being perceived as too slow. What's often overlooked, sadly, is that running can be an incredibly uplifting, sociable and inclusive activity. Running as one person in a mass of tens of thousands of likeminded souls with the same finish line in sight, can give you the biggest buzz.

Running as seen on TV and in the media often focuses on elite sport; however, it is, by virtue of its simplicity, a sport for all. It's (almost) free and can be done anywhere and at any time of life. In fact, long-distance running is thought to favour older runners who are new to the sport, basically because they usually come into running without the history of running injuries that lifelong runners may have notched up, and so they can reasonably expect to have a good few running years ahead of them.

So, what do non-runners say about starting to run? For some people, it's an activity that they just never quite managed to grasp. It never felt right. Others might feel that they'd love to run, but when they try, they can't breathe, or they get knee pain. Others say they simply have never enjoyed it. But, if we persevere and perhaps try to approach running differently, the payoff can be substantial.

Benefits of running

Running can be really good for you. Your heart gets stronger, your mind clearer and it's great for reducing body fat, if that's an issue for you. Running improves your lung capacity and strengthens your respiratory muscles. It's a weight-bearing activity, so it helps retain your bone density. Contrary to popular belief, it can help to keep joints healthy, because the muscles and connective tissue around them become stronger and this can help take the pressure off the joints themselves.

Above all this, though, running can simply make you feel better. It can give you a 'runner's high' – feel-good endorphins coursing through your veins, and then a lovely sense of calm. As it can burn fat and build muscles, running can be helpful in improving body image. It can help you concentrate afterwards, and help you sleep better that night.

A note of caution

Can I run if:

> … I'm taking Herceptin (trastuzumab)?
> … I have knee or hip problems?
> … I have cancer in my bones?
> … My breathing/swallowing is different since cancer treatment?

My answer to all four scenarios would be a cautious, qualified 'Yes, as long as…'. I've worked individually with people who've been in each of these situations, all of whom needed a little caution before embarking upon a programme of running.

Emphatically I would say to speak to your oncologist first, and, if you have access to one, a physiotherapist with oncology experience. They will be able to advise you whether your individual circumstances are such that running, for you and for now, might not be the best plan. However, if they think it would be safe, then they would be able to direct you as to how best to accommodate your current needs. So, for example, a woman on Herceptin might discuss her intention to start running at her next regular heart scan appointment, a physio might advise on gait, strength exercises and improving balance for people with joint problems or bone metastases, and a physio or SLT might be able to guide you specifically on breathing, or dealing with saliva, as you become more active.

It's important for me to say that they might recommend you *not* to run. I've been asked by several people with secondary cancer, for example, whether they're 'allowed' to run. It is possible that a clinician, if asked, will advise against it. They have good reason for this, as do clinicians in other situations. This book aims to help people make their own decisions, weighing up risks and benefits. If running is really important to you then you might decide that you're happy to do it despite the risks. I urge you to make your own informed choice.

In the four scenarios listed above I would definitely seek expert input so that you know you're doing the best thing for you, and so that you can use your clinical team's expertise to support you on your mission. Also, keep reading – Jeffing (page 119) might be for you.

How to start – Couch to 5k

I find that the best way to start, by far, is to mix brief spells of running into a longer walking session. Try jogging – slowly at first – for however long you can, whether that's 10 paces, or 1 minute, or longer. It can be 'from here to that lamp post'. As soon as you want to, take a short walking break to get your breath back. Repeat this pattern, for a total of about 20 minutes if you can. Do allow yourself walk breaks. It's not cheating.

Keep your pace comfortable. If you try to go too fast, you'll probably just hate it.

Take that first session as your baseline that you will then build on. Most training programmes suggest running three times a week, on non-consecutive days. I often use, and highly recommend, a method called 'Couch to 5k'. If you follow it, I promise you it *will* work, as long as you're consistent, but don't overdo it. There are lots of different Couch to 5k programmes, and they normally help people to train up to a point where they can run without a break for 30 minutes. There's an NHS version that you can download as an app for your phone – it talks to as you run, telling you when to take a break.

Some people want something a bit gentler than the NHS programme, and often need something that progresses more slowly and predictably week by week.

See Chapter 4 for my version of a Couch to 5k, which includes a visit every four weeks to your local parkrun (see p. 150).

How to breathe

This, for many people including me, is the deal-breaker. If you feel like you can't breathe while you're running your brain will, automatically, and quite sensibly, encourage you to stop running in order to preserve life. However, if you learn to breathe deliberately and deeply, you can control it, and stay calm and in control while you run.

Try this: jog gently and breathe in rhythm with your footsteps – try breathing in for three paces and out for three. Gently, calmly, in, two, three, out, two, three, over and over. It's up to you whether you breathe through your mouth or nose – there's no right or wrong. Play around with this rhythm until you find what feels comfortable – it might be, for example, that you prefer four paces per breath. When I'm working hard, or getting tired, I use two paces to breathe in, two to breathe out. Drop your shoulders and try to relax as you do this.

Finding and keeping this rhythm should mean that you feel more confident as you build up your running, because you can be reassured. You *can* run and still breathe. Return to this trick if you get tired but do remember that slowing down, or stopping, is always an option. You don't have to struggle or suffer in order to call yourself 'a runner'.

Run walk run – 'Jeffing'

Jeff Galloway is a running coach with the US Olympic team and a former winner of multiple long-distance races. He found that, as amateur distance running became more popular, runners increasingly were getting injured. He believed that if running was interspersed with walk breaks – like Couch to 5k – then it would be easier for the body to tolerate. He devised a method called 'run walk run', which is a formula based on your running speed and in which running is always interrupted regularly, from the start of each run, by a fast, smooth walk.

The intervals are often shorter than many people would imagine. I usually run at what he'd describe as 90:30 – I run for 90 seconds, walk for 30 seconds, for the whole of my run.

Two things are remarkable about this form of running. Firstly, you simply can go further. The constant breaks from running give your muscles a chance to work differently during the walking, and this helps them to tire less quickly. Running, broken into regular short chunks, feels less daunting too. On a longer or more challenging run, you always know that, even if you're struggling, you'll only need to run for a short time before you can recover a little during the walk section.

Some people don't get on with Jeffing – they find it interrupts their flow to be constantly changing pace. I, however, find it very rhythmic, and I feel that I can often sense when I need to change pace without having to be prompted by my watch.

The second thing about it is that, often, you'll complete a distance quicker if you 'Jeff' it than if you run constantly. I know this doesn't sound right – surely it must be slower if you're endlessly walking? Well, no, many runners find their overall speed increases. This is partly because the walk breaks allow you to risk running a little faster, safe in the knowledge that it's only for a short time. Also, part of the training is that you work on the speed of your walking, and on making your transition between walk and run smooth. I have two identical Personal Best times for the same parkrun route: one I ran constantly and the other I Jeffed.

In terms of cancer rehabilitation, this is one way into running for people with fatigue, as it's simply less daunting than attempting to run without stopping. If you're experiencing general aches and pains, but really want to run, this might work well for you (as long as it's safe for you to run). Do please check any such aches with a physio or one of your clinical team before embarking on a running programme.

You'll find Jeff at www.jeffgalloway.com.

Shoes

Wear good quality running shoes and replace them if you know they're pre-historic. There's a traditional view that trainers will give you support for around 500 miles. They don't need to be pricey, but they are your most important piece of kit. If you are going to invest in new ones, go to a running shop and ask them to do your 'gait analysis' – they'll pop you on a treadmill that has a little camera on the back, and film you as you run. (Please don't feel self-conscious here – they only film your feet and lower leg.) Gait analysis will tell you, and the shopkeeper, how you land, and what the best type of shoe is, for you.

Parkrun

Parkrun is a wonderful phenomenon that has swept across the world. It is in my view the running community at its most splendid and it is something I am personally committed to. Parkrun works like this: it's a free, timed, all-welcome 5k event every Saturday morning at 9 am. There are currently 1050 parkruns in the UK and 100 in the Republic of Ireland – find your local one at www.parkrun.org.uk/events and www.parkrun.ie/events respectively.

Parkrun is very strictly NOT a race and there are no winners – everyone completes the distance together rather than racing against each other. Faster runners elbowing slower folks out of their way is an absolute no-no. Walkers, dogs, kids and buggies are most welcome. It's not-for-profit, staffed by volunteers, and it's for everyone regardless of ability. By 10 am on Saturday morning you feel such a sense of achievement, and it's a fab way to start your weekend. It's truly a remarkable movement that has become global. Read about it and find your local one at www.parkrun.org.uk.

I think it is the ideal goal for anyone starting to run. It is habit forming, and it may well keep you on track for years to come.

5k Your Way, Move Against Cancer

Another fabulous movement that I'm proud to be a part of, is 5k Your Way, Move Against Cancer, an initiative provided by MOVE Charity. It is 'a cancer support group with a difference'. This lovely organisation does a simple yet brilliant thing – helping people affected by cancer to come together in order to take part in their local parkrun.

So, for the hesitant and the unsure, this is one way of taking part in parkrun safe in the knowledge that you will have some buddies with you who understand how much it means, for you, to be doing a 5k event at 9 am on a Saturday morning. The groups normally get together for a coffee (and perhaps cake) afterwards to swap parkrun stories. Check them out at www.5kyourway.org.

Running is a mental sport

There seems to be a symbiotic relationship between running and mental health, and there are numerous studies to show that running can help to manage depression,[19] fatigue, stress and anxiety.[20]

Running can clear your mind, certainly, and mulling over a problem can help it to ease. As you run, your mind can really wander. It can be where you do some of your best thinking, and have good, creative ideas.

For some, running can feel easier with distraction, and listening to music or a podcast can really help you to keep going. Of course, this doesn't work for everyone, and some just love the peace and simplicity of listening to what's around them, hearing the birds singing.

Gratitude

It can be really hard to push yourself out of the door to go for a run if you're feeling mentally low, or if your mojo is temporarily missing. One trick – again partly as distraction – is to try to think of things that you feel grateful for. I'm sorry – I know this might sound a little trite. And frankly if you are feeling a bit down, you might feel unable to think of much that you're grateful for at all.

But here's the thing: sports psychologists think that if you distract yourself with grateful thoughts, they will help spur you on physically. Kevin Vandi has written about this widely and says: 'Maintaining an intentional and grateful mind through training can add resiliency to hard workouts. When you're grateful for the opportunity to run, or thankful for being able to be outside safely, it makes it a little bit easier to head out when you'd rather head back to bed.'[21]

Reasons to be cheerful, it seems, include the fact that you've become a runner.

Life goals

Possibly the most beautiful run of my life was starting before dawn with a fireworks display and running into the sunrise over the Pacific Ocean – the day I ran the Honolulu marathon. It was hot, steep and stunning.

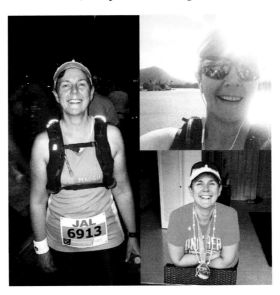

Figure 14 Running the Honolulu marathon in Hawaii

Big medal, and a big grin afterwards.

Active rest and recovery

Rest and recovery are both important aspects of a balanced, sustainable active life, and are a valid part of a training plan. When we rest, we offer our body the time to heal. Having a couple of rest days each week is a good idea and if you can build good quality rest into your routine it will serve you well both in the short and long term.

In practice it entails exercising at a less intense level than you usually would – so a gentle walk or bike ride perhaps, or some yoga or tai chi. It's when you might 'cross train' by doing a form of exercise that moves your body differently to your more regular activity. Cross training can really help with the frustration of being on the injury bench and it will contribute to getting you back in action. In the periods that I've been unable to run through injury I have often used an indoor bike instead. The trick is to make sure that the alternative exercise doesn't irritate the injury, or leave you fatigued.

Active rest helps our muscles recover.[22] It boosts circulation and helps stimulate our body's transport systems to deliver nutrients and to remove waste. Recovery time is essential when we're trying to build strength as our muscles use the rest period to adapt to the work we've asked them to do. They repair and therefore come back stronger.

A note about over-training

I know that it can be very tempting to work hard on your exercise. It can feel extra satisfying to 'go the extra mile' and it can help us to feel like we're getting back to our own normal. It can feel good to challenge ourselves.

The problem is that it can also leave us open to injury and it is horribly annoying to hurt yourself. It can undermine the gains you've worked so hard to achieve and one ill-advised move or session can take days or weeks to fix. (The irony, dear reader, is that I am writing this with one leg elevated as I have brought on a bit of 'jumper's knee' after getting carried away with a skipping rope. What a numpty.)

The need to be aware of over-training is particularly important when we think about fatigue. If we compare our energy levels to money, then if we have a big day and overspend, we have less in our pockets and have to eke out what's left till payday. A wise woman called Bernie taught me this analogy. So, I urge you to splurge sometimes, but with caution, and with a little planning so that you can have a less 'spendy' day afterwards.

So, what might the components of a rest or recovery day look like?

- **Fuel.** If you're able to, eat a mix of good quality protein (for muscle repair) and carbohydrates (to replenish your energy store).
- **Hydrate.** Water, diluted juices, electrolyte drinks if you have a stoma. Avoid sports drinks as they tend to be sugar-laden. Drink little and often.
- **Sleep.** Professional athletes need way more sleep than us mere mortals and often nap several times a day. I urge you to mimic our Olympians and have a siesta.
- **Stretch.** A slow, gentle full body stretch is a useful thing to do on a rest day – it'll help offset muscular aches or tightness. As discussed elsewhere, restorative yoga helps calm our nervous system. A massage or using a foam roller might be good too.
- **Stop.** Actually allow yourself to pause, even if it's brief. You've earnt it. I knit, with my feet up, and watch a film.

When things go wrong: what to do if you get injured

Inevitably, sometimes things go wrong, and we end up temporarily on the injury bench. When we start to exercise, or are pushing ourselves to improve, we can expect a few aches and pains. People often describe a satisfying 'good ache' a day or so after exercising.

Normally warming up diligently, and stretching afterwards, will be enough to keep everything in full working order. If you experience a mild sprain or strain, there is a method called RICE, or PRICE, that has been used successfully for decades to treat minor sports injuries.

PRICE therapy – NHS guidance

Minor injuries, such as mild sprains and strains, can often be initially treated at home using PRICE therapy for two or three days.[23]

PRICE stands for protection, rest, ice, compression and elevation.

- Protection – protect the affected area from further injury, for example, by using a support, kinesio tape or elasticated bandage.
- Rest – avoid exercise and reduce your daily physical activity. Using crutches or a walking stick may help if you can't put weight on your ankle or knee. A sling may help if you've injured your shoulder.
- Ice – apply an ice pack to the affected area for 15–20 minutes every two to three hours. A bag of frozen peas, or similar, will work well. Wrap the ice pack in a towel so that it doesn't directly touch your skin and cause an ice burn.
- Compression – use elastic compression bandages during the day to limit swelling.
- Elevation – keep the injured body part raised above the level of your heart whenever possible. This may also help reduce swelling.

If this does not work, if you are in a lot of pain or it worsens, or if you're at all worried, seek help from someone better qualified than me. Your GP, cancer team or NHS111 are there to hear from you if there is something concerning you.

Chapter 4

The practical section

Getting going

Warm-up routines

Warming up is important. It helps our heart and lungs to prepare for an increase in exertion and allows our muscles and joints to be able to move fully, with less stiffness or impingement. It needn't take long but is helpful for reducing the risk of injury.

Standing warm-up

Firstly walk or jog for 5 minutes.

Then do each of these movements 10 times – do them slowly, gently and without any force (see Figure 15).

1. Rotate each foot
2. Point your toes/flex your ankle
3. Kick each foot up behind you
4. Raise each knee in a slow march
5. Rotate each hip
6. Keeping your legs and hips still, gently twist around to each side
7. Gently bend from side to side

8. Shrug your shoulders up and down
9. Circle your shoulders forwards and backwards
10. Draw your arms across your chest.

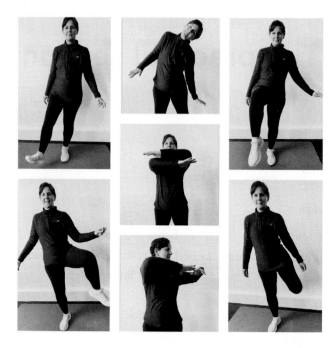

Figure 15 Standing warm-up moves

Sitting warm-up

You can do many of the warm-up moves sitting down. Begin by marching for a couple of minutes in the chair to warm up your heart and lungs (and legs). Then do each of these movements 10 times – do them slowly, gently and without any force.

1. Rotate each foot
2. Point your toes/flex your ankle
3. Raise each knee in a slow march
4. Keeping your legs and hips still, gently twist around to each side
5. Gently bend from side to side from you waist
6. Shrug your shoulders up and down

7. Circle your shoulders forwards and backwards
8. Draw your arms across your chest.

Becoming less 'chair-shaped' – sit-to-stand

Sit-to-stand is perhaps the exercise I use more than any other – it is immensely useful yet very simple. It's how Hima in Chapter 1 (page 42) got her oomph back.

Sit in a hard-seated chair that's either heavy or resting against a wall (so it can't slide backwards). Looking ahead, rather than down, stand up without pushing yourself off with your arms. Try to avoid stamping the floor – keep your feet flat, firm, hip-width apart. Sit back down again, trying to control your downward motion so that you land on the seat gently.

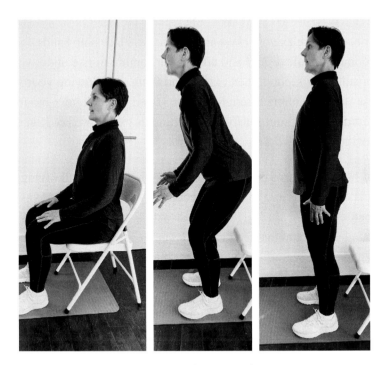

Figure 16 Sit-to-stand

Repeat this for as long as you can – 10 or 12 times might be enough for now. As you get into a rhythm, try to dig your heels into the floor when you're coming up to stand, as this activates your glutes (the big muscles in your buttocks). Gently squeeze your bum as you come to standing straight. Build this up – it'll really help. See if you can get to a point at which you can sit-to-stand for a whole minute.

Then try speeding up and work on how many you can fit in – with good technique, mind – during that minute. Eventually, it can be done holding a weight, or on one leg.

How to breathe more easily

Reminding ourselves how to breathe deeply and rhythmically can make moving feel much more manageable. Try the following exercise.

Lie on your back and relax your chest and shoulders. Place both hands lightly on top of your abdomen. Inhale deeply and allow your tummy to rise under your fingers. Hold the breath for a second, then exhale and focus on allowing your stomach to fall. Practise deep breathing through your nose and through your mouth. Practise concentrated deep breathing for five to 10 minutes each day. Try it in a sitting or standing position when working on other tasks.

Next, learn how to control the rhythm of your breathing. While lying or sitting, do a few relaxed breaths as above. Now count as you breathe: inhale as you count to three, then exhale for three. (I've started with a count of three, but do choose whatever number to count that feels right for you.) Get used to this sense of rhythm, in and out, and count according to however you feel most comfortable.

We can play around with the rhythm of our breathing, according to the activity we are involved in. Yoga practice can include lengthening our exhalation, so we keep breathing out, slowly and steadily, until our lungs feel fully emptied. This might involve a rhythm where breathing out lasts twice as long as breathing in. It's important to note that this should always feel comfortable – you shouldn't find yourself lengthening a breath only to find you're gasping for air.

One breathing exercise that can feel even more calming is to exhale through your mouth, slowly and steadily, with your lips pursed, as if you're blowing through a straw.

After thinking about how we breathe when we're motionless, we can progress to work on breathing while moving – for example, try breathing in for a count of three and out for a count of two. This method is used by running coaches to help athletes keep a sense of control as they push themselves to run faster.

To do this, start by breathing in a 3:2 rhythm whilst standing up – then progress to tapping alternate feet to the rhythm, breathing in for three taps, and out for two. Now try walking, using that rhythm but taking one step rather than a tap and so that one round of breathing in and out is spread over five steps. It's up to you whether you breathe through your mouth or nose – there's no right or wrong. Some people find that when they exercise, they prefer to inhale through their nose and exhale through their mouth.

Synchronising the rhythm between your breaths and steps should mean that you feel more confident, and that your breathing stays controlled as you climb stairs. This method of breathing can be used in lots of circumstances, and I've used it many times to help people who are learning to increase the intensity of their exercise routine.

Make the stairs part of your exercise plan

When you're ready to, add into your daily routine a stair climb, where you purposefully breathe well. Stand tall with your chest open and shoulders back, and practise climbing the flight with as much control as you can. Count how many steps you can manage before needing to hold the banister and then challenge yourself to make the point that you hold on gradually higher up than previously. Channel Sylvester Stallone doing Rocky's stair climb, complete with theme tune, if it'll help.

If you don't feel ready to tackle a whole flight of stairs, step on and off the bottom step of a flight of stairs. Do as many step-ups as you can and then rest.

Try to gradually increase the number of steps that you can do before you need to stop.

Want to make stair climbing feel easier instantly? Try planting your whole foot on each stair, rather than stepping on your toes. Then press down firmly through your heel as you bring your body weight upwards. This will activate your gluteal (buttock) muscles and allow the strength that you already have in them to propel you upwards.

Pelvic floor exercises

Now, for this I need to call a spade a spade...

You can do this standing, sitting or lying down. Imagine you are right in the middle of urinating and you need, for whatever reason, to suddenly stop the flow. Squeeze the little muscles that you'd use to stop peeing. Hold them for a few seconds and then gently release them.

This is a specific, localised movement and nowhere else should move – not your buttocks, legs, or your tummy muscles or your face. Learn how to find those muscles and contract and release them. Try it a few times until you're confident that you can squeeze then release on demand. (This should mean that you've got more control if you are about to sneeze or cough etc.) Then try holding the squeeze for a little longer before you release. Make sure that you keep breathing naturally throughout. Do this regularly, several times a day.

Also try working on your 'back' muscles: imagine you are trying to stifle an urge to pass wind. Again, squeeze the muscles that you'd need to use to do that. They're not the same as the first ones. Squeeze and contract, several times, and for differing amounts of time. Make sure you don't move your buttocks or thighs – it's another really tiny movement.

With both sets of muscles, try training them to do 10 squeeze-then-release exercises, then try doing 10 where you hold for a little longer, then 10 where you do quick, fast pulse-like squeezes. Try to teach the muscles to do a 'pyramid' squeeze – first

1 out of 10 in terms of grip, then 2, 3, 4, building up gradually until you squeeze at full 10 out of 10.

Getting out of puff

Chair-based cardio

At its gentlest, you can follow this routine by focusing movement on your legs, swinging your arms by your side. The intensity of the exercise will be greater if you also do the arm movements or make each move larger. This can be increased further by holding a small hand weight, wrist weight, tin of beans etc.

This works best in a chair that is comfortable, wide enough for you to move in, and that is stable enough that it won't tip backwards or roll away from you. If you're in a wheelchair or a seat with casters, put the brake on. It should be high enough that you can sit with your knees at an angle of about 90 degrees, but not too high – you need your feet to be flat on the floor. Arm rests can offer a bit of support if your energy is low, but you may find you need to lower them or move to a chair without arm rests if they impede your full movement.

Do as many of each move as feels right for you. Be mindful of any injuries that you're currently experiencing, especially in the shoulders or back. Perhaps start with 12, or 20 repetitions, or time yourself – maybe do 30 seconds of each and take a break in between moves. You can adapt this totally to your own energy levels each time. This works really well with music as the beat will help you find your rhythm.

Throughout this routine, try to sit up tall with your back straight and your shoulders relaxed. Lean on the back of the chair if you want it to support you – but if you can manage without it you'll give your belly and back muscles more work to do.

Warm up first, then:

1. March in the chair (Figure 17), whilst bending the opposite arm.
2. Knee lift with bicep curl (Figure 18). A slower bigger march, bending both arms at the elbow.

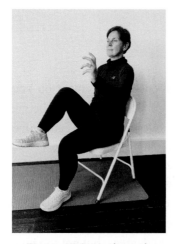

Figure 17 Seated march

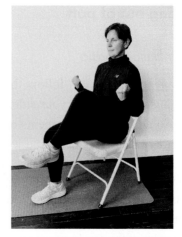

Figure 18 Seated knee lift and bicep curl

3. Toe tap and chest press (Figure 19). Reach out each foot and tap the floor in front. Push both arms forwards.
4. Heel tap and triceps press (Figure 20). Reach out each foot and tap the heel. Drive your arms backwards, as if you were skiing.

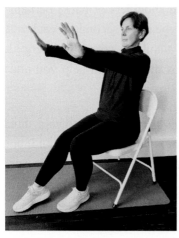

Figure 19 Seated toe tap and chest press

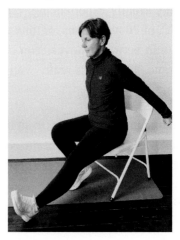

Figure 20 Seated heel tap and triceps press

5. Marching arm scissors (Figure 21). March in the chair. Swing one arm up in front of you and the other back behind your hip.

6. Heel raise and throw (Figure 22). Bounce your heels up and down whilst throwing an imaginary ball over your head.

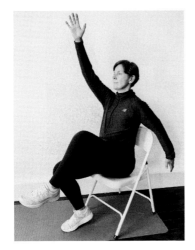
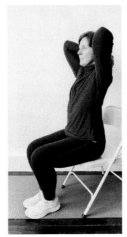
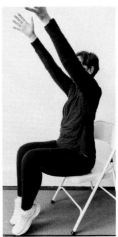

Figure 21 Seated chair arm scissors   Figure 22 Seated heel raise and throw

7. Marching X (Figure 23). March, and make an X shape with your arms – above your head, back to your belly then down by your hips.

8. Tap and reach (Figure 24). Tap your right foot out to the right whilst swinging your right arm overhead. Repeat on the left.

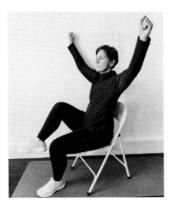
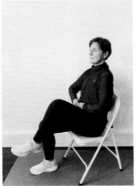
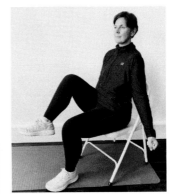

Figure 23 Seated marching X

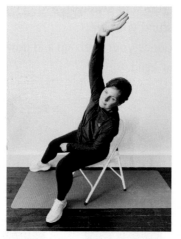
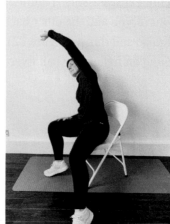

Figure 24 Seated sidewards toe reach

9. Seated star jump (Figure 25). Keeping your back straight and long, hop both feet out, arms wide, in and out.
10. Sit-to-stand (see Figure 16, page 42). In a chair that can't rock or slide backwards, stand up, keeping both feet flat on the floor, then sit down, trying to keep your knees pointing forwards as you move.

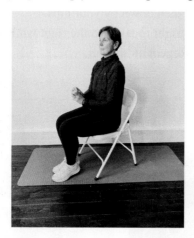
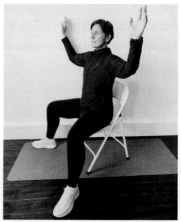

Figure 25 Seated star jump

Repeat the whole routine if you have the time and energy.

Roger's dining table routine

This is the routine that Roger and I used to do, around his dining table, performed to one of his favourites – Ella Fitzgerald, singing *Mack the Knife*. It's gentle and, if you use the same song, takes 4 minutes. It can be performed using a resistance band tied around your legs (underneath your kneecaps) for added oomph. All the moves are illustrated in figures in this chapter.

- Verse 1: Step to the side – eight in one direction, eight back (see Figure 69)
- Verse 2: hamstring curls (see Figure 60)
- Verse 3: fire hydrant (see Figure 59)
- Verse 4: heel raises. On both feet, bring your heels up so that you are standing on the balls of your feet, then slowly lower back to the ground. Don't let your ankles roll inwards or outwards as you do it
- Verse 5: knee raises (see Figure 70)
- Verse 6: gentle squats – we would only go halfway down (see Figure 27)
- Verse 7: march on the spot
- Verse 8: crab walk (see Figure 56).

Weight-bearing, no-equipment cardio training

I recommend you start with the low impact version of this routine. Take your time as you familiarise yourself with the moves and try to do them with really good posture.

Use the higher impact version if you want to bounce more, but please read the cautions relating to specific side effects or conditions as they apply to you – especially around recent surgery, bone metastases, back issues and hernia risk.

Warm up first and then do a round of each of the moves listed in Table 6 – my suggestion is to start with 10 or so of each exercise, having a short rest in between. Alternatively, time yourself – 30 seconds on each move is a good starting point.

Table 6: Weight-bearing exercises

Low impact	Higher impact/intensity
1. March on the spot	1. Jog on the spot
2. Wall press (Figure 26a). Stand on the balls of your feet facing a wall with your hands on the wall at shoulder height and width. Without bending your hips or spine, dip your face towards the wall by bending your elbows and shoulders.	2. Press up (Figure 26b). Same as the wall press but on the floor, on your hands and knees. Remember there should be no bend in your spine or hips. If you're strong enough, you could do a full press up with hands and feet on the floor.
3. Squat (Figure 27a). With your feet hip-width apart, toes facing forwards, squat, as if you're about to sit on a chair. Your bodyweight should move backwards, and your shins stay vertical. Don't let your knees move forwards. Stand up, driving your heels into the ground as your rise.	3. Squat with knee drive (Figure 27b). As you rise out of each squat, drive one knee up high. Alternate sides.
4. Walk and punch (Figure 28a). March forwards, and back, punching straight in front of you.	4. Jog forwards and back, punching straight in front. Try punching above your head for added oomph (Figure 28b).
5. High knees. March on the spot, bringing your knees up as high as you can.	5. High knees. Jog on the spot, bringing your knees up as high as you can
6. Half star (Figure 29a). Tap your right foot out to the right while bringing the opposite arm out wide. Repeat on the left.	6. Star jumps (Figure 29b). Jump both feet apart whilst swinging your hands up towards your ears. Jump back to standing position and lower your arms.
7. Side-step to wide squat (Figure 30a). Take three wide steps to one side then squat down with your feet at shoulder width, then three steps back and repeat on the other side.	7. Side shuffle touch floor (Figure 30b). Take three bouncy steps to one side. Looking forwards and keeping your back straight, touch the floor then repeat on the other side.

(Table continues on page 144.)

(a)

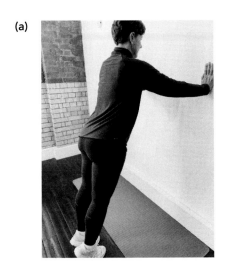 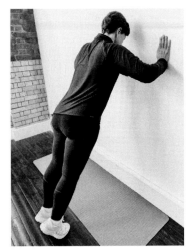

(b)

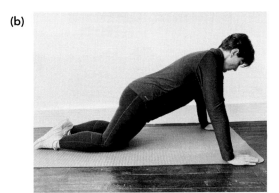

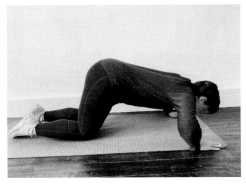

Figure 26(a) Wall press; (b) Press up

(a)

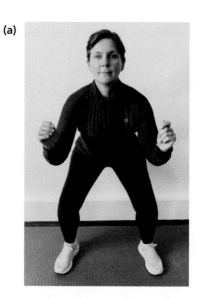

(b)

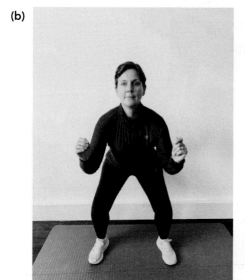
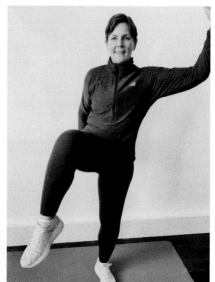

Figure 27(a) Squat; (b) Squat with knee drive

(a)

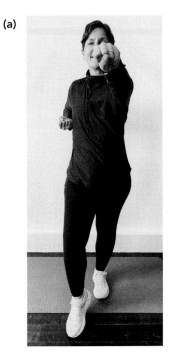

(b)

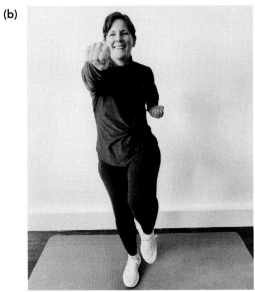

Figure 28(a) Walk/punch; (b) Jog/punch

(a)

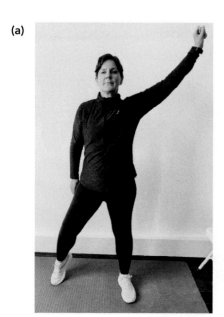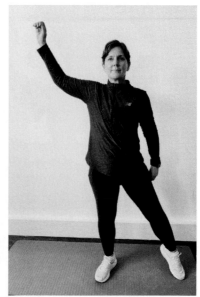

(b)

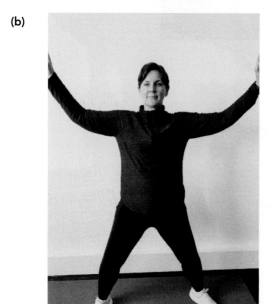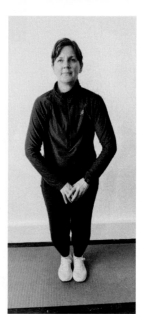

Figure 29(a) Half star; (b) Star jumps

(a)

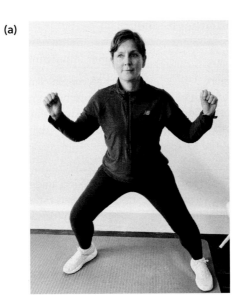

(b)

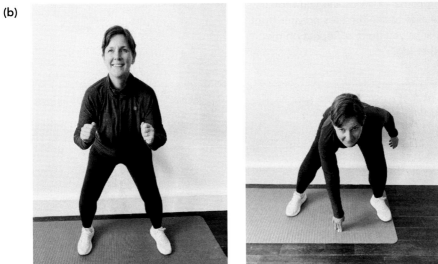

Figure 30(a) Side-step to wide squat; (b) Side shuffle touch floor

Table 6: Weight-bearing exercises (cont'd)

Low impact	Higher impact/intensity
8. Mountain climber (Figure 31). Supporting yourself on a chair, stretch out straight so there's no bend in your spine or hips. Bring your right knee up towards your right elbow and repeat on the left.	8. Mountain climber – faster. Try doing these but moving your feet more quickly. Make sure you hold your posture – don't let your back bend.
9. Back lunge (Figure 32a). Using a chair or rail for support if you want it, take a really big step backwards. Then bend both knees, sinking your body down vertically. Make sure you bend both knees equally – this should feel like your back leg is working harder than the front. Your front knee should not come forwards and you should be able to see the toes on your front foot as you do this. Repeat on the other leg.	9. Walking lunge – lunge by stepping forwards rather than backwards, moving forwards with each one (Figure 32b).
10. Fast feet – march on the spot as quickly as you can.	10. Fast feet – jog on the spot as quickly as you can.

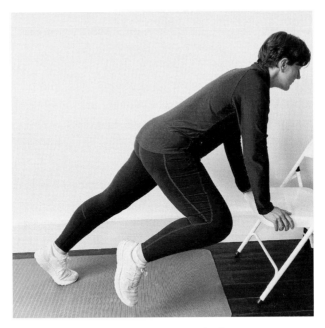

Figure 31 Mountain climber

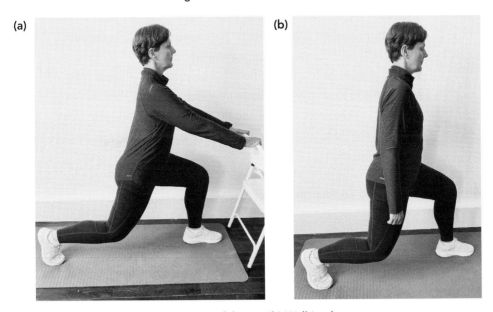

Figure 32(a) Back lunge; (b) Walking lunge

Exercising without squishing the belly

This is a good routine for anyone worried about leakage.

1. Get out of puff… Walk tall, with good posture, and with purpose – this should be brisk but comfortable, as if you are marching. Walk quickly enough so that you are a bit out of breath. Make it strenuous to challenge you, but not so much that it becomes daunting. Aim for 20–30 minutes a day.
2. Get strong. Do strength training two to three times a week, on non-consecutive days.

    a. Follow the upper body exercises later in this chapter (page 151).
    b. For your lower body: squats (see Figure 27) – but if you're worried about leaking, do them with your feet wider apart. Do some with your toes pointing forwards, and some plié squats with your toes at an angle of 45 degrees.
    c. **Glute bridge** (see Figure 50), crab walk, fire hydrant and hamstring curls (see Figures 56, 59 and 60) all avoid squashing the bladder.
    d. **Mountan climber** (see Figure 31) – taking the knee outwards in a wide diagonal line rather than towards the chest.
    e. For the core muscles, pelvic floor training, pelvic tilt and TVA hold are a good place to start and to build confidence from. They're described in detail in 'Getting going' at the beginning of this chapter (page 127) and the core strength part of 'Getting strong' later in this chapter (page 151).

Step-by-step guide to Nordic walking

1. Nordic walking poles are different to hiking poles, and they are designed to allow your hands and shoulders to move fully. Their height should be set so that, if you stand up with your elbows tucked into your waist, and hold the handle, your forearm is parallel with the ground (Figure 33a).
2. The straps should be tight enough that they won't slip off, but loose enough that you can comfortably move your wrists. You hold the poles by

curling your fingers around the pole. Your grip needs to be gentle but firm (Figure 33b).

3. You start by walking naturally with the poles simply trailling behing your feet (Figure 33c). Posture should be good, standing upright, shoulders back and arms relaxed. Walk as briskly as you comfortably can.

4. As you walk your arms swing by your side – if they don't do this naturally then don't worry. Don't overthink this. As each arm swings backwards with your step, press the pole down and back into the ground, pressing through the palm of the hand into the cloth of the strap. Push down *and* back so you feel the floor/ground disappearing away from you – this is how it works – you push down and back and the poles propel you up and forwards.

5. Get used to how this feels, walking with your arms in rhythm with your feet (this can take a little while), and giving the pole a little push down and back with each step (Figure 33d).

6. Then, try to make the movement a little bigger, by slightly picking up the pole with each step before gently hitting the ground and pushing it down and back (Figure 33e). You don't need to lift it much at all, just enough that it leaves the ground. It should then hit the ground by your foot and not in front of it.

7. Think about how your arm swings: Nordic walking technique asks you to move your whole arm from the shoulder, rather than the elbow (Figure 33f). The elbow stays soft and your movement all comes from the shoulder. It looks very much like the way a soldier would march. It can take a little time to learn this but it's worth it as it helps with shoulder strength and range of movement.

8. Think about how you're using your feet and, if you can, try to roll your bodyweight from your heels through to the balls of your feet, as if the soles of your feet are curved. You'll utilise the strength in your feet and calf muscles better and might feel a little more bounce with each step.

9. As you become more familiar with Nordic walking, try pushing your hand backwards a little further, past your hip, so that your arm's stride becomes

a little longer (Figure 33g). Nordic walking should feel purposeful and your arms feel active and engaged.

10. As you get to grips with step 9, try to slightly open and close your fingers at the very end of each push on the poles (Figure 33h). This will be more comfortable for your wrists, and it's one of the ways in which using the poles helps us to manage lymphoedema – that gentle pulsing of the fingers encourages lymphatic drainage.

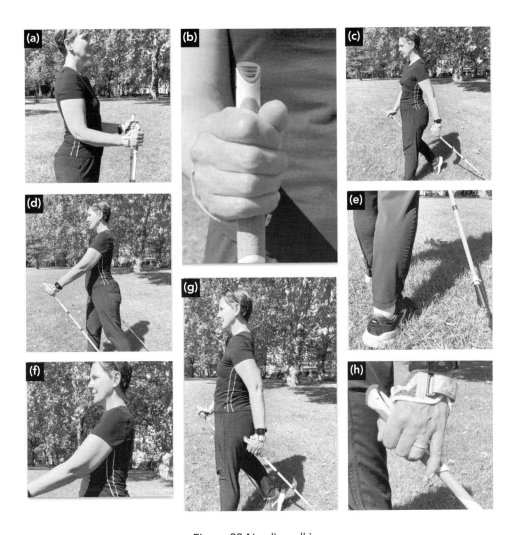

Figure 33 Nordic walking:

(a) pole height; (b) grip poles; (c) poles trail behind; (d) pole pushed down and back;
(e) pick up pole; (f) move from the shoulder; (g) past your hip; (h) open and close fingers

Couch to 5k plan: walk, jog or run

Train three times a week – try Tuesdays, Thursdays and Saturdays. All sessions begin with a 5-minute walk to warm up, and end with a 5-minute cool down walk.

Do repeat the current week or go back a week if you need to – this is *your* plan. Then move on when you're ready.

Go at a pace at which you're out of puff, but can still talk, even if it's just in short phrases rather than long sentences. If you're struggling, slow down.

This plan works equally well as a walking plan as one for running – use the intervals marked 'run' to walk as fast as you can and the 'walk' sections to go at your regular walking pace.

Table 7: Twelve-week 'Couch to 5k' plan

Week	Activity
1	Run 30 seconds, walk 30 seconds x 15
2	Run 45 seconds, walk 45 seconds x 15
3	Run 60 seconds, walk 60 seconds x 15
4	Do a Saturday parkrun. Run and walk as much as feels comfortable Rest of the week: run 90 seconds, walk 60 seconds x 12
5	Run 2 minutes, walk 1 minute x 10
6	Run 2.5 minutes, walk 1 minute x 9
7	Run 3 minutes, walk 1 minute x 8
8	Do a Saturday parkrun. Run and walk as much as feels comfortable Rest of the week: run 3.5 minutes, walk 1 minute x 7
9	Run 4 minutes, walk 1 minute x 7
10	Run 4.5 minutes, walk 1 minute x 6
11	Run 5 minutes, walk 1 minute x 5
12	Do a Saturday parkrun – try to run the whole way, taking a short walk break after every km. Have a couple of rest days before you plan your next challenge.

Getting strong

Exercises to improve upper body strength, using a resistance band

1. **Banded chest press** (Figure 34). Wrap the band around your back and hold it underneath your armpits with your elbows bent and fists facing side on. Slowly straighten your arms, then return them to the starting position.
2. **Lateral pulldown** (Figure 35). Hold the band, moderately taut, above your head with your hands at shoulder width. Gently lower your arms, drawing your hands wider as they lower – each hand will travel in a diagonal line.

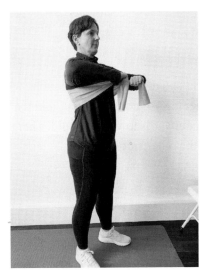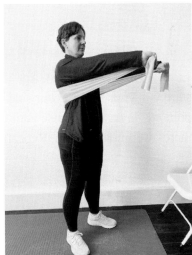

Figure 34 Banded chest press

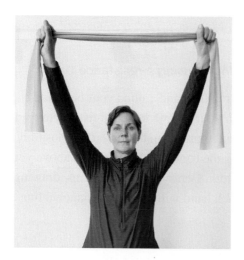
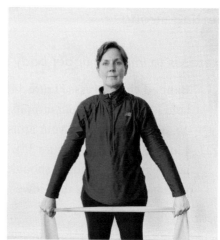

Figure 35 Lateral pulldown

3. **Lateral raise** (Figure 36). Anchor the end of your band under one foot and start with your arm by your side. Keeping your arm straight, and the thumb pointing downwards, raise your arm outwards towards shoulder height and then lower it back down. Repeat on the other side.

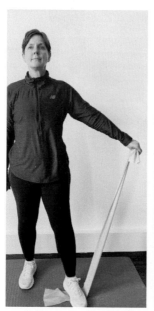
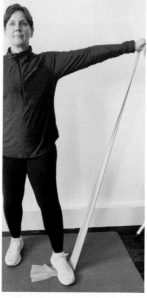

Figure 36 Lateral raise

4. **Triceps press** (Figure 37). Hold one end of the band behind your head and catch hold of the other end by the base of your spine. Slowly straighten your upper arm, stretching the band upwards. Make sure the band stays in a straight line and follows the middle of your back and head.

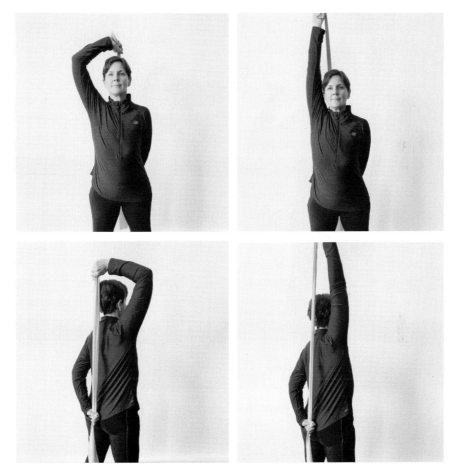

Figure 37 Triceps press

5. **Shoulder press** (Figure 38). Secure the end of the band under one foot, and at full length with your fist by your armpit. With your palm facing away from your body, stretch your arm straight up as far as you can above your head, keeping the rest of your body still. Then do the same on the other side.

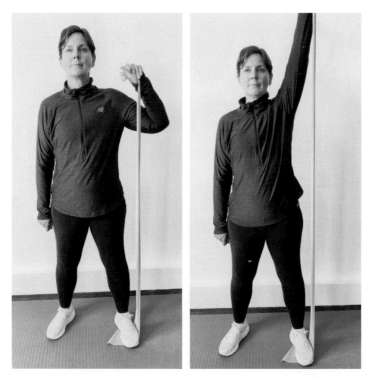

Figure 38 Shoulder press

6. **Banded row** (Figure 39). Anchor the middle of the band securely around a door handle, post etc. Hold your tummy muscles taut and the band in each hand with your elbows bent and by your waist. Draw your elbows and shoulder blades back, in a rowing motion. Don't rock the rest of your body – only your arms should move.

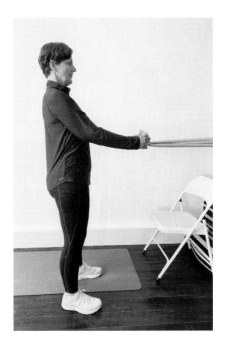 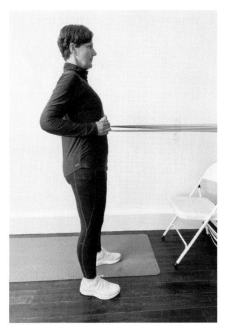

Figure 39 Banded row

7. **Upright row** (Figure 40). Stand with one foot in front of the other, and the middle of the band under your front foot. Hold your fists together in the middle of your tummy. Draw your hands gradually up the middle of your torso with your elbows wide – the movement should start in your shoulders and upper arms, rather than your elbows. Draw your arms upwards until your fists are up to your armpits (no higher). Your elbows should be higher than your fists the whole time.

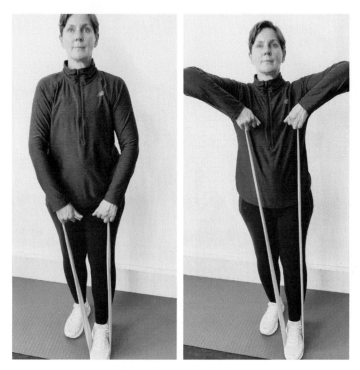

Figure 40 Upright row

8. **Wall press** (See Figure 26a). Stand on the balls of your feet facing a wall with your hands on the wall at shoulder height and width. Without bending your hips or spine, dip your face towards the wall by bending your elbows and shoulders. If this feels too easy, try taking a tiny step further away from the wall, drop your hands a little lower so they're still at shoulder height, and try this again.

9. **Front raise** (Figure 41). Anchor your band under your left foot and hold the band in your left hand in front of you, fist around hip height, with your arm straight (elbow is soft). Lift your arm until your fist is as close to shoulder height as you can. When you're doing this, try to keep your body still, avoiding the temptation to rock backwards. Then do the same on the right.

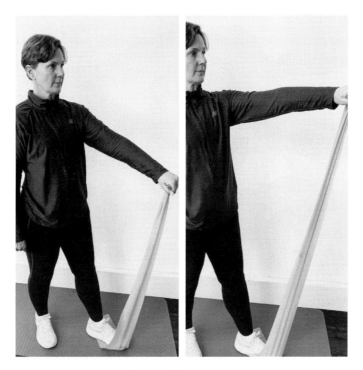

Figure 41 Front raise

10. **Chest fly** (Figure 42). Drape the band over the back of your shoulders, so that it's resting on the inside of your elbows, and not up near your neck. With your elbows soft, draw your arms out as wide as you can, and then, without bending your elbows, bring them together out in front of you.

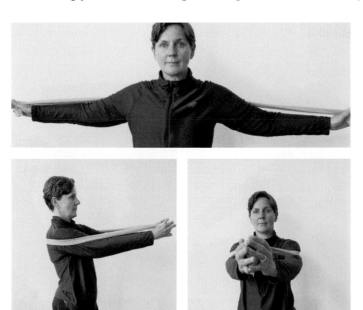

Figure 42 Chest fly

Strength training with a Hickman or PICC line or Portacath

Here are three useful upper body strength exercises that should feel fine. Before you start, it's worth doing some small gentle movements (reaching upwards, pushing outwards, raising your arms out to the side etc) just to reassure yourself that the line/port feels secure as you move.

1. **Banded row**. Anchor a band securely in the middle around a door handle, post etc. Hold your tummy muscles taut and the band in each hand with

your elbows bent and by your waist. Draw your elbows and shoulder blades back, in a rowing motion (see Figure 39).

2. **Banded chest press**. Wrap the band around your back and hold it underneath your armpits with your elbows bent and fists facing side on. Slowly straighten your arms (see Figure 34).

3. **Lateral raise**. Anchor the band under one foot. Keeping your arm straight, raise your fist up to shoulder height and lower (see Figure 36). Repeat on the other side.

This is deliberately a very cautious and short list as I'm keen to avoid risking injury. Once you feel confident, (and by all means check in with your clinical team first) then start to look at the general upper body exercises, beginning with small versions of each and using only your bodyweight before you try adding any resistance. Build up very gradually and stop if you think the exercises are causing the line/port to move or feel unstable.

Strength training for those with lymphoedema

One starting point for these exercises is to do some good, deep, relaxed breathing, where you send your inhaling breath to your belly rather than holding it in your chest. This is recommended prior to exercising and before manual lymphatic drainage, as a way of gently stimulating the lymphatic system.

It's important to warm up before starting, so move a little before doing these exercises – march on the spot, walk around the garden etc for a few minutes.

On the next pages are exercises for the upper body, legs and groin, and head and neck; they are intended for anyone experiencing lymphoedema as well as being at risk of it. At level 1 these are gentle pumping motions in which you'll move your muscles and joints, but without any resistance, to help stimulate the lymphatic system.

Once you're comfortable with, and not challenged by, level 1, move on to level 2, in which you may start to build strength. (You could still perform level 1 as your warm-up first.)

Upper body strength for lymphoedema – level 1

These exercises are to be performed initially by just using your body weight, and with your hands empty.

Start with five relaxing deep breaths, then perform five of each of these:

1. **Jazz hands**. Make a fist, then splay your fingers widely (Figure 43).
2. **Flex wrists**. Keeping your elbows still and by your ribs, roll your fists up and down (Figure 44).
3. Shrug your shoulders up towards your ears, then drop them down, as low as is comfortable.
4. Try also the lateral raise, triceps press and shoulder press described earlier in this chapter (Figures 36, 37 and 38) and the arm movements shown in the chair-based cardio exercises (Figures 17–25). Begin with just your body weight.

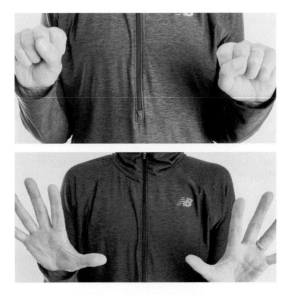

Figure 43 Jazz hands

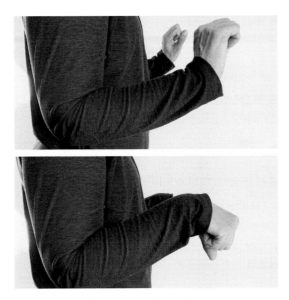

Figure 44 Flex wrists

Do this sequence a few times and, when you're ready, gradually increase the number of repetitions of each exercise until you're comfortable doing 12 or more.

Upper body strength for lymphoedema – level 2

Once you've got used to level 1, move on. Although it's important to build up gradually, you do want to move onwards and upwards once you're ready, otherwise your strength will plateau. You may find that level 1 is too gentle immediately.

So, try doing the same exercises, but with some added resistance. Start with a light hand weight, wrist weight or resistance band. Tins of beans or small plastic water bottles also work well. Instead of 'jazz hands', try gently squeezing a tennis ball.

You want to be using enough resistance so that your muscles start to tire after 10 or 12 repetitions of each exercise – this might take a little guesswork at first, as you're going to start again with just five repetitions but, if in doubt, start light then build up. If you're experiencing peripheral neuropathy in your hands, you could try using small wrist weights that fasten lightly around the wrist with a Velcro strap if your grip's not so good.

Level 1 exercises can be done every day. Once you start to move on to level 2, my recommendation is to do level 1 as a warm-up first. Level 2 should be done on non-consecutive days, ideally three times a week, as part of your muscular strength building.

Strength training for lower limb lymphoedema – level 1

Start with five deep breaths and, using just your bodyweight for now, do five of the following – the ankle pumps (Figure 45), knee bends (Figure 46) and leg extension (Figure 47) shown here, and the leg curl and knee raise seen later in this chapter (see Figures 57 and 70).

1. **Ankle pumps**. Point your toes, then flex your ankle (Figure 45).

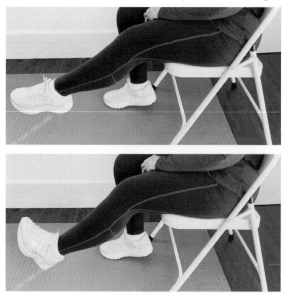

Figure 45 Ankle pumps

2. **Knee bends**. Bend and straighten the knee (Figure 46).

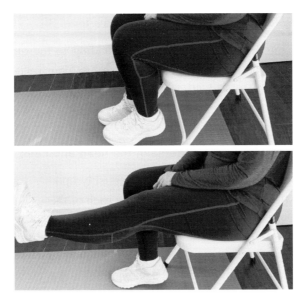

Figure 46 Knee bends

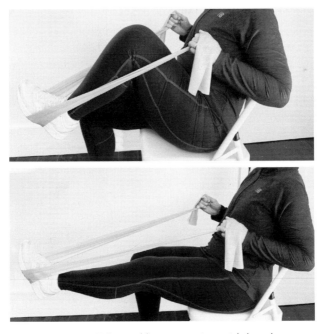

Figure 47 Seated leg extension with band

Strength training for lower limb lymphoedema – level 2

As before, once you're ready to move on, try adding in the other moves in the lower body strength routine on p. 172–178. Use just your own body weight for the exercises at first, then gradually start adding resistance with a light weight or resistance band.

Stretches for those with lymphoedema in the head and neck

The following are exercises recommended to assist lymphatic drainage around the head and neck. After your deep breaths, try five each of these (Figure 48):

- gently bring your chin down towards your chest, then tip your head to one side then the other
- roll your shoulders forwards and backwards then, keeping them still, gradually turn your gaze over one shoulder then the other.

Also try the shoulder shrug listed in the warm-up routine for the upper body at level 1 (see p. 160).

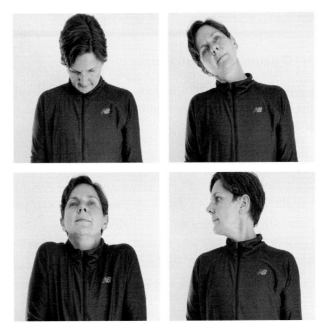

Figure 48 Neck and shoulder stretches

Afterwards, do some deep, diaphragmatic breathing, drink water and, if you can, make a little time to relax. You might (literally) put your feet up for a few breaths: if you're comfortable doing it, lie on your back with your bottom near to a wall and the soles of your feet up on the wall, legs straight upwards.

Strength training after breast reconstruction

Exercising after reconstruction with implant(s)

In the first six weeks after breast reconstruction, concentrate on your upper body mobility exercises. After this time, it is usually advised to be safe for you to return to 'normal activities', but you should avoid lifting heavy weights. I recommend you start to build upper body strength using the routine earlier in this chapter (see p. 151). Perform your mobility exercises first each time, as a warm-up, and then, using a very light resistance band at first, start building up. Ideally, do upper body strength training two to three times a week on non-consecutive days. And do, absolutely start light and then build up slowly. It's fine also to exercise your abdominal muscles.

Stay aware – nothing should hurt and if it does, stop.

Exercising after LD (latissimus dorsi) flap

Reconstruction that utilises fat, skin and (in the case of TRAM) muscle from elsewhere in the body is a little more complex, and takes longer to heal and, therefore, to rehabilitate.

With LD flap, you need to avoid any form of resistance completely for six to eight weeks after surgery, and from then on, the best advice is that it's okay to start to lift things that are 'slightly heavier'. At this point (and no sooner), you could start to perform upper body strength moves with the lightest resistance band, again going back over your mobility exercises as a warm-up. You could also begin to exercise your abdomen and back. As with an implant, the best outcomes are seen if these exercises are done two to three times a week and, again, please don't overdo it. Be slow, deliberate and progressive.

With an LD flap, around 12 weeks post-surgery you could start – gradually, of course – to increase resistance.

Exercising after TRAM and DIEP flaps

Reconstruction that involves the abdomen requires a little more caution and consideration. TRAM (transverse abdominis myocutaneous) flap carries a risk of hernia, DIEP (deep inferior epigastric perforators) flap less so as it doesn't involve the abdominal muscles. For either, a period of at least seven weeks is recommended before any training at all, and please bear in mind that it can take six to eight *months* before the abdomen feels as supple as it was prior to reconstruction.

You should avoid all abdominal exercises until after seven weeks. Around this time you could begin working your upper body – with the same cautions as above: nothing should hurt, start light and increase the amount of effort involved very slowly and deliberately. Be a stickler for good technique. The following are recommended as ways to begin to train your trunk, or core muscles, after DIEP or TRAM.[1]

Exercising after TRAM/DIEP – level 1

Start with:

1. **Pelvic tilt** (Figures 49a and 49b). Taking care not to move your thighs, knees or buttocks, tuck your tail bone under so you feel your tummy muscles tighten and a stretch in your lower back. Try to move only the muscles in your trunk and not your legs.

(a)

(b)

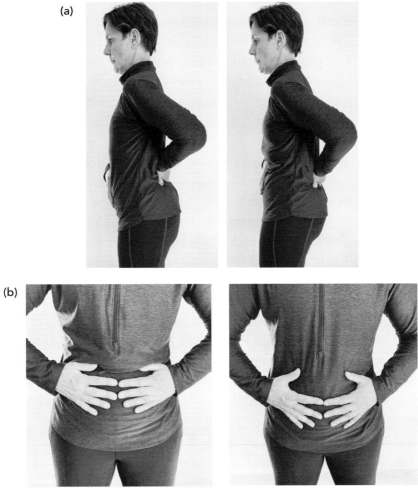

Figure 49(a) Pelvic tilt side view; (b) Pelvic tilt – hands

2. **TVA hold.** The transverse abdominis (TVA) is sometimes referred to as a natural corset, or natural 'spanx' – and if you were wearing a very big pair of knickers, they'd cover it. The TVA is a large sheath of muscle that runs around our torso and it is a crucial part of our core strength. It is what protects the spine and keeps it stable when we move our limbs. There is no illustration here, because, and as with pelvic floor exercises, there's nothing to see. There should be little discernible movement therefore this is an exercise that you can do anywhere and people won't know you're doing it: Sit comfortably or stand with a neutral spine, feet flat and weight evenly distributed. Take a good deep breath and, as you exhale, pull your tummy muscles in, as if you're trying to pull your bellybutton towards your spine. Hold that position while you begin to count (in your head or out loud). Don't hold your breath though – you're trying to hold just the muscles in a brace-like hold, not your breath. Start by holding and counting to 3 and then build up.

3. **Glute bridge** (Figure 50). Lying on your back with your feet up by your bum, very slightly tuck your tailbone underneath you, so there's no arch in your lower back. Holding that position, raise your hips upwards. You don't need to go too far for this to work – and make sure you avoid exaggerating the move so much that your back bends. Hold the position at the top for one breath, then lower. Try to keep your knees pointing forwards, rather than them falling inwards as you move.

4. **Pelvic floor exercises** (using them here for their help in overall core strength, rather than specifically around incontinence, see p. 132).

5. Add in some **seated toe taps** – sitting tall, reach out with one foot then the other and tap the floor in front of you (see Figure 19). Make this a small movement at first but build up until you can reach out with the foot until your knee straightens. Try to hold your back long and tummy muscles taut as you do these.

6. **Hip flexor stretch**. Gently stretch your hip flexors (Figure 51).

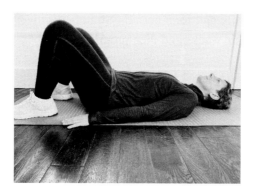

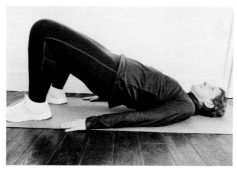

Figure 50 Glute bridge

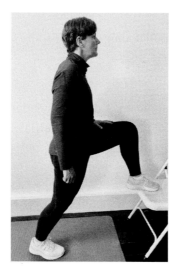

Figure 51 Hip flexor stretch

You could do these daily and for a period of time – it's a very personal choice but I'd allow a month or six weeks and then progress.

Exercising after TRAM/DIEP – level 2

This involves adding a little more body weight into each move. Try the following:

- **Bird dog** (Figure 52). From all fours, reach your right leg and left arm in straight lines away from you. Try to keep your back straight and still – don't roll your hips or shoulders. This is a move where you try to lengthen, rather than lifting your limbs upwards. Return to the starting position and repeat on the other side.
- **Dead bug** (Figure 53). Lie on your back with your arms up straight, and your legs up, but with your knees bent, shins parallel with the floor. Position your spine so it's 'neutral' – not arched or rounded, but comfortable. Then, without letting that spinal position change, simultaneously lower your right arm over your head and your left foot towards the floor. Return them to the starting position then work the opposite limbs. (If this feels too intense, try a half dead bug – holding the legs in the starting position whilst moving each arm, or hold the arms still and move the legs.)
- Try the chair-based routine on p. 133 for some safe cardio exercise.

Exercising after TRAM/DIEP – level 3

Again, in your own time (but again, I'd recommend a few weeks) proceed to the 'gentlest' variations of core strength exercises seen later in this chapter (see Figures 62a to 67a).

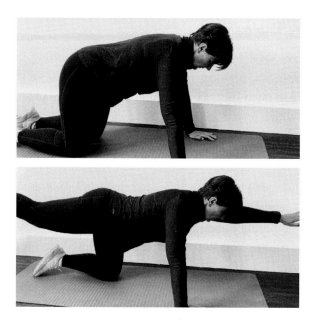

Figure 52 Bird dog

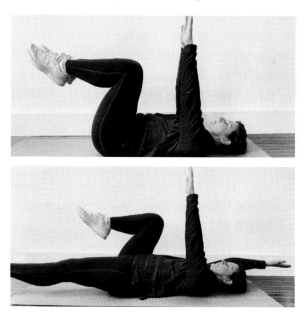

Figure 53 Dead bug

Lower body strength training

As with other exercises, I recommend beginning by learning how these moves should look and feel and perform 10–12 of each one. If you've got the energy, do them all, have a rest, then repeat the routine. Some of these just use body weight, others are better with a resistance band.

The most useful exercises for lower body strength, I believe, are:

1. **Sit-to-stand** (see Figure 16). In a chair that can't rock or slide backwards, stand up, keeping both feet flat on the floor, then sit down, trying to keep your knees pointing forwards as you move.
2. **Squat** (see Figure 27a) With your feet hip width apart, toes facing forwards, squat, as if you're about to sit on a chair. Your bodyweight should move backwards, and your shins stay vertical. Don't let your knees move forwards. Stand up, driving your heels into the ground as you rise.
3. **Back lunge** (see Figure 32a). Using a chair or rail for support if you want it, take a really big step backwards. Then bend both knees, sinking your body down vertically. Make sure you bend both knees equally – this should feel like your back leg is working harder than the front. Your front knee should not come forwards and you should be able to see the toes on your front foot as you do this. Repeat on the other leg.

These make a great basis for any strength programme. Add in exercises that train our muscles differently, such as:

1. **Plié squat** (Figure 54). Like a regular squat but starting with your feet really wide and at a 45-degree angle. As you squat, make sure you sit back, rather than letting your knees sink forwards.

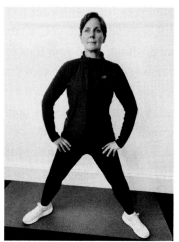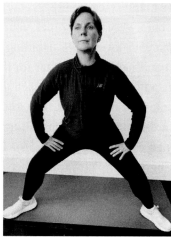

Figure 54 Plié squat

2. **Wall sit** (Figure 55). Lean against a wall, with all of your spine and shoulders touching it. Bend your knees, sliding down it until your thighs are horizontal – make sure your feet are far enough from the wall that your shins can be vertical. Hold for as long as you can.

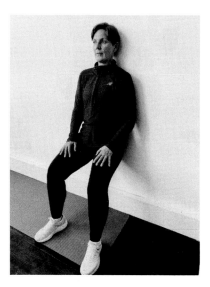

Figure 55 Wall sit

3. **Glute bridge** (see Figure 50). Lying on your back with your feet up by your bum, very slightly tuck your tailbone underneath you, so there's no arch in your lower back. Holding that position, raise your hips upwards. You don't need to go too far for this to work – and make sure you avoid exaggerating the move so much that your back bends. Hold the position at the top for one breath, then lower. Try to keep your knees pointing forwards, rather than them falling inwards as you move.

4. **Banded crab walk** (Figure 56). Take wide steps sidewards. Move by cocking your hip upwards rather than reaching or scraping your foot along the floor. Make this harder by tying a band around your legs (but not touching your kneecaps).

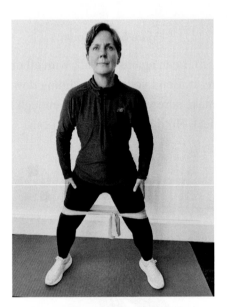

Figure 56 Banded crab walk

5. **Seated leg extension** (see Figure 47). This works best with a resistance band. With the band securely around the arch of one foot (not on your toes – it'll ping off), draw that knee towards your chest. Straighten your leg by stretching the heel out in a horizontal line.

6. **Banded leg curl** (Figure 57). Tie a band around the ball of one foot and then draw the band, and your foot, back towards you. Without lifting your thigh, gently straighten your leg by curling the foot upwards. Then repeat on the other side.

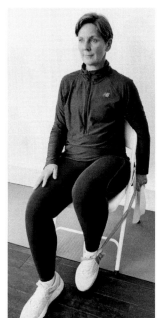 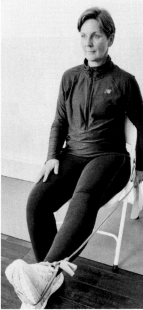

Figure 57 Banded leg curl

7. **Glute kickback** (Figure 58). Tie a resistance band around both ankles and then move your foot so that the band sits around the arch of your right foot, bending your right knee towards your chest. Then straighten the leg out behind you, moving your foot away in a horizontal line. Try to move the working foot parallel with the ground rather than swinging it upwards. Repeat on the left.

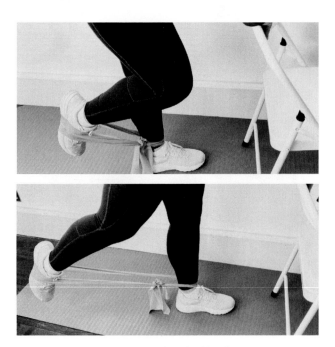

Figure 58 Glute kickback

8. **Banded fire hydrant** (Figure 59). Keeping the rest of your body still, cock your leg, just like a dog might. Try adding a band above or below the knees.

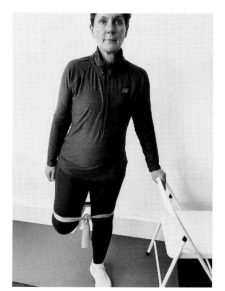 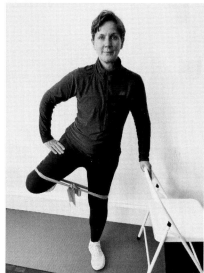

Figure 59 Banded fire hydrant

9. **Banded hamstring curl** (Figure 60). Without letting your working knee move forwards, scoop one foot up behind you as if you were trying to kick your own bottom. Try adding a band around the ankles.

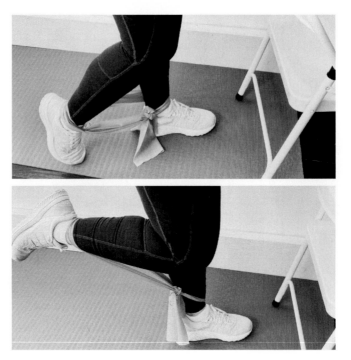

Figure 60 Banded hamstring curl

Back and core strength exercises

The foundation of good strength training for your belly and back should, I believe, begin with three key moves: Pelvic tilt, TVA hold and Pelvic floor training. I strongly recommend that, whatever your starting point, begin by getting to grips (literally!) with these.

1. **Pelvic tilt** (see Figures 49a and b). Taking care not to move your thighs, knees, or buttocks, tuck your tail bone under so you feel your tummy muscles tighten and a stretch in your lower back. Try to move only the muscles in your trunk and not your legs.

2. **TVA hold**. As mentioned earlier, the transverse abdominis (TVA) is sometimes referred to as a natural corset, or natural 'spanx' – and if you were wearing a very big pair of knickers, they'd cover it. The TVA is a large sheath of muscle that runs around our torso and it is a crucial part of our core strength. It is what protects the spine and keeps it stable when we move our limbs. There is no illustration here, because, and as with pelvic floor exercises, there's nothing to see. There should be little discernible movement, therefore this is an exercise that you can do anywhere, and people won't know you're doing it. Sit comfortably or stand with a neutral spine, feet flat and weight evenly distributed. Take a good deep breath, and as you exhale, pull your tummy muscles in, as if you're trying to pull your bellybutton towards the spine. Hold that position while you begin to count (in your head or out loud). Don't hold your breath though – you're trying to hold just the muscles in a brace-like hold, not your breath. Start by holding and counting to 3 and then build up.
3. **Pelvic floor training** – there's a detailed description of these on page 132 – see the section on 'getting going'.

As with other exercises, please note any specific restrictions or side effects that apply to you. There's a range of exercises here so if you know you need to avoid certain moves – such as sharp bends or twists of the spine – then there's still plenty to be getting on with. If you have a hernia or hernia risk, remember – exhale as you exert. These exercises ask a lot of the muscles, so I'd start with perhaps six of each and build up from there. Do as many as feels right for you and stop if anything feels uncomfortable.

Paying close attention to good posture and technique, try these:

1. **Bird dog** (see Figure 52). From all fours, reach your right leg and left arm in straight lines away from you. Try to keep your back straight and still – don't roll your hips or shoulders. This is a move where you try to lengthen, rather than lifting your limbs upwards. Return to the starting position and repeat on the other side.

2. **Superman** (Figure 61). Lying on your tummy, lift your right arm and left leg gently off the floor. Keep your head in a neutral position, looking downwards. You might feel the muscles along your spine working. Depending on your flexibility, this can be a small move – it shouldn't feel uncomfortable at all. Hold for a couple of seconds then lower back to the floor. Repeat on the oposite side.

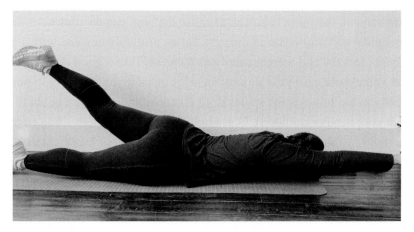

Figure 61 Superman

3. **Dead bug** (see Figure 53). Lie on your back with your arms up straight, and your legs up but with your knees bent, shins parallel with the floor. Position your spine so it's 'neutral' – not arched or rounded, but comfortable. Then, without letting that spinal position change, simultaneously lower your right arm over your head and your left foot towards the floor. Return them to the starting position then work the opposite limbs. (If this feels too intense, try a half dead bug – holding the legs in the starting position whilst moving each arm, or hold the arms still and move the legs.)

The next set of back and core strength exercises in Table 8 are given in two versions, so you can progress to greater intensity when you feel ready.

Table 8: Gentle and more intense back and core strength exercises

Exercise	Gentlest	Progress to...
Abdominal crunch. Lie on your back with your knees bent and spine neutral. Slowly lift your chin and chest upwards (don't bend your back). The backs of your shoulders will lift a little off the floor (Figure 62a)	Slide your hands up towards your knees (Figure 62a)	Lift a little higher so that your shoulder blades leave the floor (Figure 62b)
Knee lifts. Sit up tall with your spine neutral. Without arching or rounding your back, lift one knee, then the other. The movement should be smooth, not jerky	Single seated (Figure 63a)	Double (Figure 63b). Once this feels comfortable, try lifting both knees together
Adapted plank. Support your upper body on a chair or bench, resting on your hands. Stretch out so your spine is straight and hold for as long as you can. Keep your neck in a neutral position and don't let your hips sink or your back bend. Your belly might wobble	Elevated, straight arms (Figure 64a)	Elevated, on forearms (Figure 64b)
Side bends. Without rocking forwards or backwards, gently bend to one side then the other	Body weight (Figure 65a)	With a band (Figure 65b)
Bicycle twist. Sitting or standing tall with your back straight, move one elbow towards the opposite knee, meeting in the middle so they almost touch if you can. Try to really open your chest as you return to the starting position	Seated (Figure 66a)	Bigger move, standing (Figure 66b)
Adapted shoulder tap. Adopt plank position but with your feet hip width apart. Gently transfer your body weight onto one arm so that you can tap your shoulder with the other. Try to do this without moving your spine	Elevated touch shoulder (Figure 67a)	Elevated reach in front (Figure 67b)

NB: Several of the upper body exercises also help to strengthen the back muscles.

See also the sections on exercising with ostomies, avoiding hernias and pelvic floor training in Chapter 1.

(a)

(b)

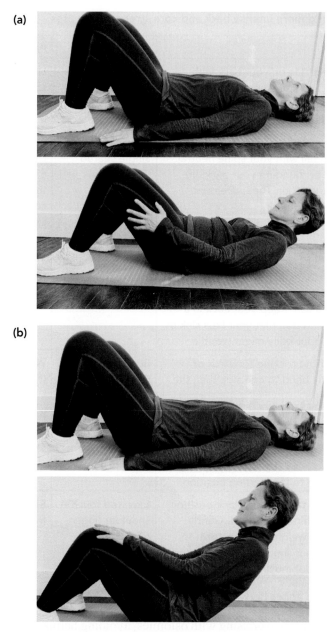

Figure 62 Abdominal crunch (a) gentlest; (b) progress

(a)

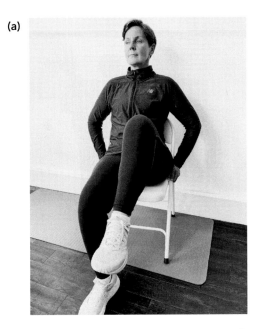

(b)

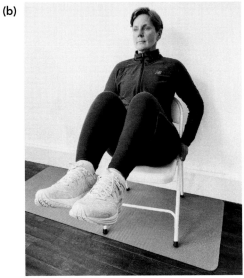

Figure 63 Knee lift (a) gentlest; (b) progress

(a)

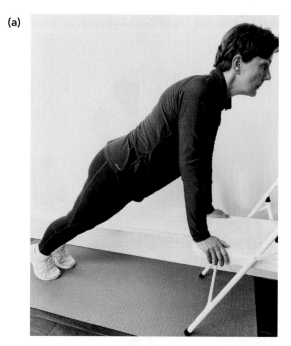

(b)

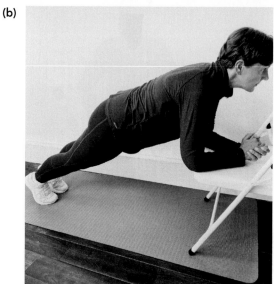

Figure 64 Adapted plank (a) gentlest; (b) progress

(a)

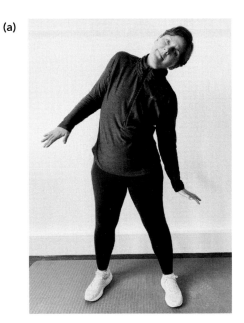

(b)

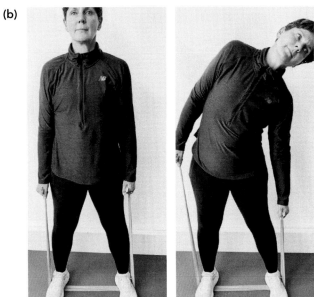

Figure 65 Side bends (a) gentlest; (b) progress

(a)

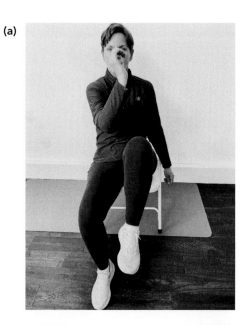

(b)

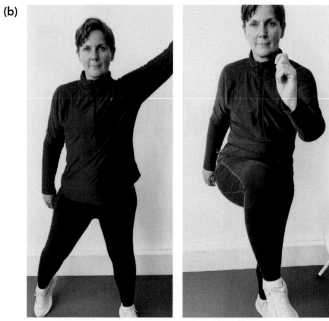

Figure 66 Bicycle twist (a) gentlest; (b) progress

(a)

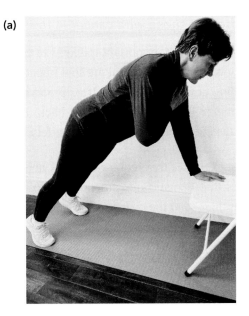

(b)

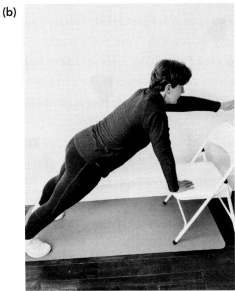

Figure 67 Adapted shoulder tap (a) gentlest; (b) progress

Core strength exercises for those with cancer in the bones/spine

As outlined in Chapter 2, it's really important to exercise in ways that will reduce the risk of fracture, so look for activities that are low impact and non-contact, and with attention on reducing any risk of falling. It is important to protect the spine, so avoid sharply twisting or bending/arching your back, and plan strengthening exercises that work on the back and tummy muscles safely.

 The trick is to focus on exercises that require the back and torso to remain stable as opposed to exercises that demand movement – for example, bring the knees towards the chest rather than bend the chest towards the knees.

Here are some exercises that you could try:

- Pelvic tilt, TVA hold and pelvic floor exercises described opposite and on pages 132–133. They're a really good foundation.
- Adapted plank (see Figure 64a and 64b). Support your upper body on a chair or bench, resting on your hands. Stretch out so your spine is straight and hold for as long as you can. Your belly might wobble.
- Mountain climber (see Figure 31). From plank position, gently bring one knee up towards your chest, or towards the same elbow. Try to do this without moving your back, staying in plank position. Repeat on the other foot.
- Try the knee lifts and toe taps described in the seated cardio routine on page 134. If these feel ok to you, try doing the whole routine.
- Roger's dining table routine on page 137 is safe and short – helpful if you're low on energy and using music may well boost your mood.
- The upper body strength routine on page 151 should be fine for you but do start with a really light resistance band to avoid putting too much load on the tendons and ligaments that are part of how we move our bones.
- The lower body strength routine (see page 172) also could work well for you but I would avoid the glute bridge as it may put pressure on your spine if you bend your back as you lift your hips.

If you experience any increase in bone pain, report it to your clinical team.

Strength training with an 'ostomy'

Please read the section on 'ostomies' in Chapter 1 before trying any of these – I want you to feel safe as you begin to exercise and there's some information there to help build confidence.

Breathe out each time you work your abdominal muscles: exhale as you exert. These moves should not cause any pain, especially in the abdominal region or in your back. If they do, stop, and discuss how it felt with one of your clinical team.

Some gentle moves to begin with are:

- **TVA (Transverse abdominis) hold**. Sit comfortably or stand with a neutral spine, feet flat and weight evenly distributed. Take a good deep breath and, as you exhale, pull your tummy muscles in, as if you're trying to pull your bellybutton in all the way to your spine. Hold that position while you begin to count out loud. Don't hold your breath though – you're trying to hold just the muscles, not your breath; this is why we start by counting out loud – it's difficult to hold your breath if you're speaking. Start by holding and counting to 3 and then build up.
- **Pelvic tilt** (see Figures 49a and 49b). Taking care not to move your thighs, knees or buttocks, tuck your tail bone under so you feel your tummy muscles tighten and a stretch in your lower back. Try to move only the muscles in your trunk and not your legs.
- **Glute bridge** (see Figure 50). Lying on your back with your feet up by your bum, very slightly tuck your tailbone underneath you, so there's no arch in your lower back. Holding that spinal position, raise your hips upwards. You don't need to go too far for this to work – and make sure you avoid exaggerating the move so much that your back bends. Hold the position at the top for one breath, then lower. Try to keep your knees pointing forwards, rather than them falling inwards as you move.

Start by doing six or so of each move – do please stop if anything hurts or feels uncomfortable. You could do these exercises every day until they no longer challenge you. Build up gradually until you can do 10 or 12 of each exercise, and then introduce some of the 'gentlest' section of the core training exercises earlier in this chapter into your routine.

Exercises to improve balance

Do these exercises as slowly as you can and don't worry if you wobble – that's supposed to happen.

1. **Stand on one leg** (Figure 68). Try circling each arm as you do this, then circle each leg. See if you can make the circles bigger and/or slower.

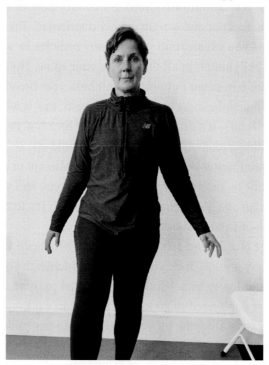

Figure 68 Stand on one leg

2. Take **slow side steps** – whilst looking ahead (Figure 69).

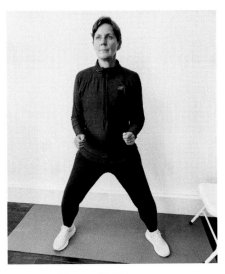

Figure 69 Side steps

3. **Slow knee raises** (Figure 70). Try reaching both arms up.

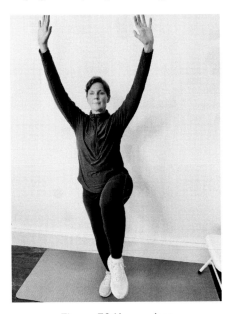

Figure 70 Knee raises

4. **Grapevine** (Figure 71). Step sideways by crossing one leg behind the other.

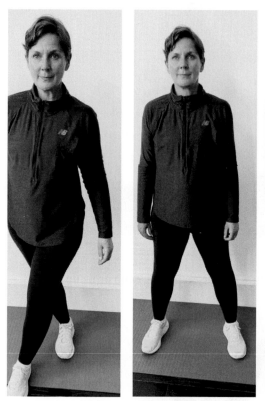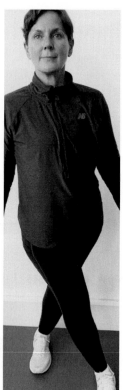

Figure 71 Grapevine

5. **Slow step up** (Figure 72). Try adding in a knee lift.

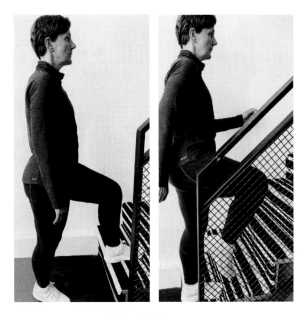

Figure 72 Step up

6. **Heel-to-toe walking** – as if you're on a tightrope (Figure 73). Do this looking ahead. Try going backwards. If you're feeling brave, try doing it with your eyes closed.

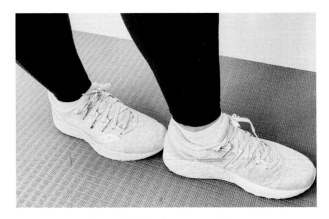

Figure 73 Heel-to-toe walking

7. **Tree** (Figure 74). Rest one foot against your knee, then slowly bring your arms above your head. Repeat with the other foot.

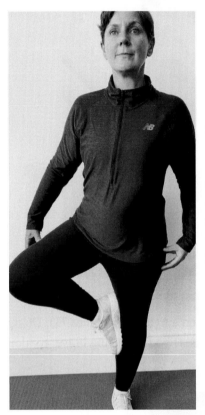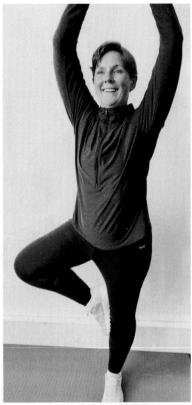

Figure 74 Tree

Full body stretch

These stretches should feel pleasant and not painful. Hold each one for 10–20 seconds – or longer if you've time. Hold the position still – don't bounce, and don't overstretch. Perform each exercise on both arms/legs.

1. **Calf stretch** (Figure 75). Supporting yourself on a chair, take a big step backwards. With your front knee bent and back knee straight, press your back heel into the floor.

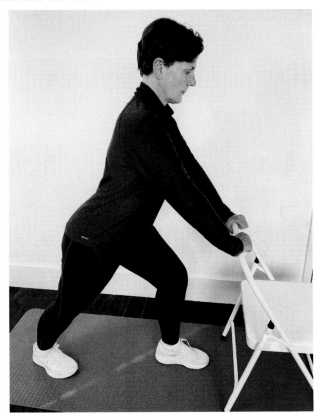

Figure 75 Calf stretch

2. **Hamstring stretch** (Figure 76). Elevate one foot on a chair or step. With both knees soft, reach your chin and chest forwards (not down), slightly arching your back. Then repeat with the other foot.

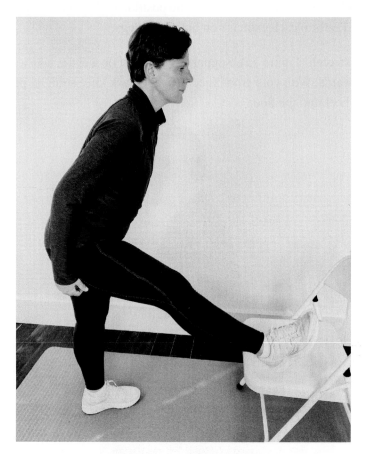

Figure 76 Hamstring stretch

3. **Quadriceps stretch** (Figure 77). Hold one foot behind you (or elevate it behind you on a chair or step). Stand tall, with your knees close together. Then repeat with the other foot.

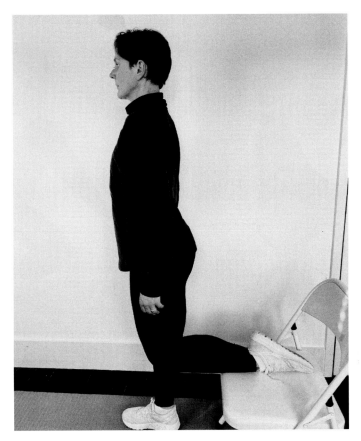

Figure 77 Quadriceps stretch

4. **Glute stretch** (Figure 78). Hold one knee up towards your chest. If you're able to, also try to balance your ankle on the opposite thigh, gently bending the knee on your standing leg. For this it may help to support yourself with one hand on the back of a chair. Then repeat on the other side.

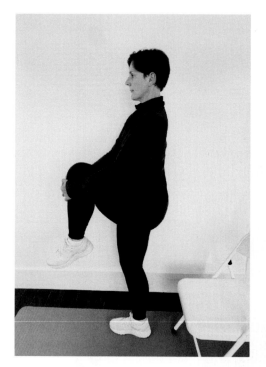 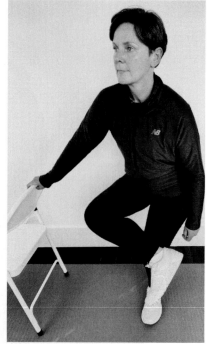

Figure 78 Glute stretch

5. **Mid-back stretch** (Figure 79). Sitting down, lean your left elbow on your left thigh and then reach your right arm forwards and then over to the left, stretching your ribcage. If you can keep your hips still whilst doing this, you should feel a stretch also in your mid/lower back. Repeat with your left arm forwards.

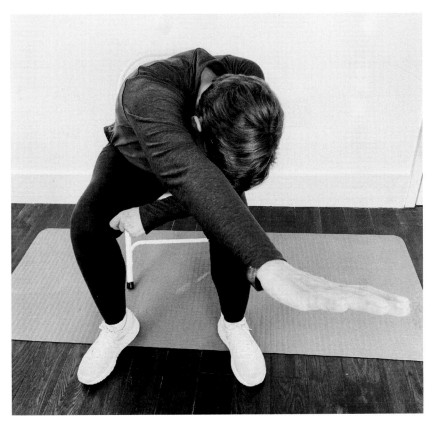

Figure 79 Mid-back stretch

6. **Back of shoulder stretch** (Figure 80). Bring one arm straight across your chest then guide it nearer to your body with the other arm. Repeat with the other arm.

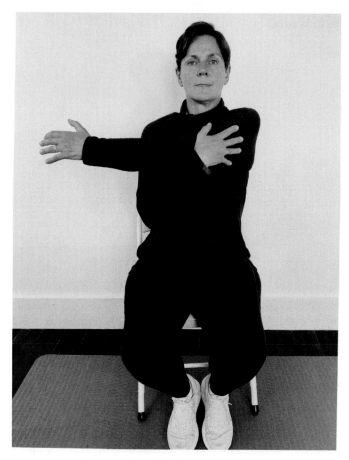

Figure 80 Back of shoulder stretch

7. **Triceps stretch** (Figure 81). Bend one arm at the elbow then raise it up and outwards, as far as is comfortable. Repeat with the other arm.

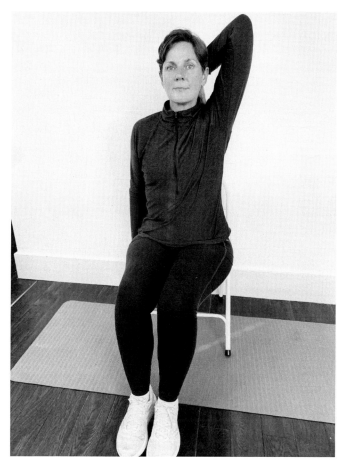

Figure 81 Triceps stretch

8. **Front of shoulder stretch** (Figure 82). Reach both hands behind you, clasp them together, then drop your shoulders.

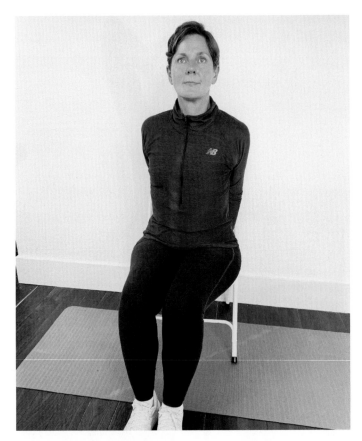

Figure 82 Front of shoulder stretch

9. **Lower back stretch** (Figure 83). Lying on your back, bring your knees to your chest then gently hug them.

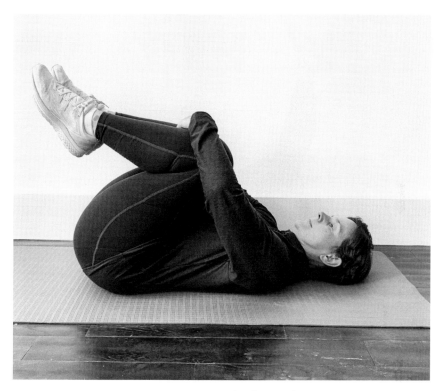

Figure 83 Lower back stretch

10. **Hip stretch** (Figure 84). Lying on your back, bend one knee towards you and then bring the other leg up behind it, to act as a lever.

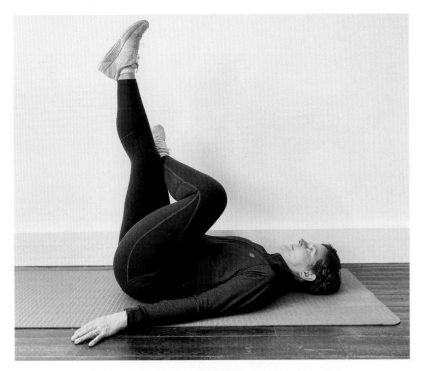

Figure 84 Hip stretch

Appendix

Cancer support organisations

I hope that this book has got you well on your way to happily and confidently being active in ways you can enjoy for good. Here are some organisations in the UK and elsewhere that I've personally dealt with over the years and which have cancer-specific, life-affirming services that you may enjoy. I heartily recommend them all. On pages 205–210 I have also included organisations in the Republic of Ireland specifically.

- **5k Your Way, Move Against Cancer**. 'A support group with a difference.' Meet up with other folks affected by cancer and take part – run, jog, walk or volunteer – in a local parkrun. Really friendly groups, all very welcome. Find them here: https://5kyourway.org/
- **Active Ostomates**. Free exercise sessions, online and through local support groups, for people living with a stoma. A brilliant range of activities from chair yoga to a 50k challenge and some team sports as well as activities for individuals. Find them at www.colostomyuk.org/active-ostomates/
- **After Breast Cancer Diagnosis**. ABC Diagnosis is an organisation and network offering peer to peer support for people with breast cancer, run by a wonderful woman called Jo Taylor. She runs residential exercise and wellbeing retreats and is currently training other women to be Nordic walk leaders. There's also an impressive online library of information. ABCD are here: www.abcdiagnosis.co.uk
- **Canrehab Trust**. Launched in 2020, this charity has developed a register of approved personal trainers and health professionals qualified to provide

tailored exercise programmes for people with cancer. Find them here: www.canrehab.co.uk/canrehab-trust

- **Dragonboat racing**. Dragon boat racing for women after breast cancer started in Canada thanks to a clever chap called Dr Don McKenzie who spotted the myriad potential benefits of team-based rowing. It's now a worldwide phenomenon with crews across the USA, Canada, Australia, South Africa, New Zealand, Ireland, Singapore, Italy, Poland as well as several in the UK. A lovely combination of effective outdoor exercise and peer support. Find refence to one near you here: www.wikipedia.org/wiki/Breast_cancer_survivors%27_dragon_boating#Dragon_boat_festivals

- **Indy SurvivOars** – boxing and rowing. This organisation caught my eye because they mix dragon boat racing with boxing as a group – these women punch 100-lb bags for fun! Interesting and forward thinking to use boxing in this way. They're based in Indiana. Read about them here: https://blog.thebreastcancersite.greatergood.com/cs-boxing-as-healing/

- **Macmillan Move More**. Macmillan Cancer Support have been at the forefront of exercise and cancer in the UK for several years. Their Move More campaign includes DVDs, booklets and online resources that you can download, plus a broad range of in-person exercise groups and classes. There's absolutely loads of good stuff – start here: www.macmillan.org.uk

- **Maggie's Cancer Support Centres**. 'Just walk in.' A charity very close to my heart – it's a privilege to work for them. Maggie's provide wonderful, broad support for anyone affected by cancer. As well as emotional, practical and financial support, most Maggie's centres run exercise sessions in-person and online. Find them here: www.maggies.org

- **Move Charity** provide practical and online support for children and young people living with and beyond cancer. As well as starting the 5k Your Way, Move Against Cancer initiative (open to all ages), this charity has a wide range of online exercise and support services. www.movecharity.org

- **Movember**. It started as a call to grow a 'tache during November as an awareness campaign around men's cancers but the charity is now focusing on helping men with prostate or testicular cancer to get moving through their MOVE campaign. Find the bro's at www.uk.movember.com/programs/inactivity

- **Nordic Walking UK/British Nordic Walking**. If I've whetted your appetite for Nordic walking, these two organisations can put you in touch with a local instructor who will normally offer a free taster session. Find them at www.nordicwalking.co.uk/ and www.britishnordicwalking.org.uk/. Beyond the UK, see the International Nordic Walking Federation: www.inwa-nordicwalking.com/

- **Nutrition**. Good diet and exercise, when combined, should bring your oomph back quickest. BUPA in the UK have a helpful guide to nutrition during and after treatment: www.bupa.co.uk/health-information/cancer/eating-well-cancerLikewise,the Cancer Support Community, based in California, have some useful advice: www.cancersupportcommunity.org/article/diet-nutrition-cancer-survivors

- **Odyssey** takes people (over 18) on a five-day residential journey to combat the psychological and emotional effects of their cancer, helping them to rebuild their confidence, engage with exercise and take back control of their lives. It is based around outdoor adventure activities and is free of charge. It is currently available in Kent and Scotland but plans to expand further. Find them at: www.odyssey.org.uk/

- **The Ostomy Studio**. Fellow cancer rehab instructor, fellow author and complete expert in her field, Sarah Russell has established a unique in-person and online range of services to help those with a stoma to safely and effectively become more active. Find Sarah here: www.theostomystudio.co.uk

- **Ovacome**. Online exercise sessions for women with ovarian cancer (plus loads of other specific support and information. Find it here: www.ovacome.org.uk/event/gentle-home-exercise-class

- **Team Phoenix Foundation**. Team Phoenix support women to train for their first triathlon after breast cancer. Seriously. www.teamphoenixfoundation.co.uk

- **Trekstok**. Trekstok offer support to anyone diagnosed with cancer in their 20s and 30s. Loads of support available here, exercise and otherwise, including their fabulous RENEW programme and a range of online classes: www.trekstok.com.

- **Vicky Fox Yoga**. Vicky's cancer-specific yoga classes are legendary in West London and rightly so. They're a really lovely way to press your 'reset' button. In person and online. You can find her here: www.vickyfox-yoga.com/about

I wish you every success, and hours of fun, getting your oomph back.

Other ways to get your oomph back in Ireland

- **5k Your Way, Move Against Cancer** are linked to parkrun in Ballincollig (Cork), Oranmore (Galway), Tralee (Co Kerry) and Marlay and Porterstown in Dublin. Find them here: www.5kyourway.org
- **ARC Cancer Support** provides services free of charge to anyone affected by cancer as well as their loved ones, and they are currently running physiotherapy-led online exercise classes. More information, and some useful info about exercising at home, can be found at: www.arccancersupport.ie/services-for-you/classes
- **ExWell Medical** offers community-based supervised exercise classes, home-based programmes and online exercise classes to people with many different long-term illnesses. Many of their classes are free of charge. You can find them at: www.exwell.ie
- **Get Active After Cancer** is an exercise programme that helps men to get active after a cancer diagnosis, run by Cork ARC, in partnership with the Mardyke Arena UCC. https://corkcancersupport.ie/get-active-after-cancer-2
- **Irish Cancer Society** have a whole range of support and services for folks with a cancer diagnosis, including some home based exercises here: www.cancer.ie/cancer-information-and-support/staying-well-while-staying-home/home-exercises-for-cancer-patients-and-survivors
- **OpFit** prehabilitation programme is the first pre-operative exercise programme for patients who are scheduled for cancer surgery in Ireland and is based at St James's, Dublin. Since the coronavirus pandemic

they have offered zoom-based exercise sessions. For more information on the OpFit programme, please contact physiotherapist Sarah Moore (0874001157, samoore@stjames.ie)

- **Pink Ribbon Pilates** – six week pilates programmes for women after breast cancer surgery, based in Dublin. www.pinkribbonpilates.ie
- **Purple House Cancer Support Centre** in Bray, Co Wicklow, has a superb cancer rehab gym, plus counselling and therapy rooms, a children's sensory pod and therapy room, cancer survivorship classrooms, a coffee dock, a drop-in facility and a therapy garden. For more information, please visit: www.purplehouse.ie or call 01-2866966.
- Rehab for prostate cancer in Waterford. Keep an eye on this one, fellas. Waterford Institute of Technology and the UPMC Hillman Cancer Centre at the UPMC Whitfield Clinic in Waterford are conducting research aimed at developing an effective rehabilitation programme for prostate cancer patients. The research will run during 2021.
- **Row to Recovery** is a river-based rowing charity based in Galway, started by three women recovering from breast cancer and a volunteer coach. It's now open to men and women diagnosed with any cancer. If you fancy a row on the river Corrib, contact them at: www.rowtorecoverygalway.ie
- **St James's Hospital, Dublin**. The Oncology Physiotherapy team provides both an inpatient and outpatient service to patients referred by their Consultant teams. The team includes a clinical specialist working in prehabilitation to prepare patients living with cancer for surgery. Both senior and staff grade physiotherapists work in cancer rehabilitation, helping patients to live during and after cancer treatment.
- **Siel Bleu**. Although not exclusive to cancer, Siel Blue is a not-for-profit organisation that provides life-enhancing exercise programmes, with the aim of improving overall wellbeing. It runs community-based programmes, one-to-one exercise programmes, and free online exercise classes – there's an extensive library of sessions on youtube, here: www.youtube.com/user/SielBleuIreland. More information about the organisation is here: www.sielbleu.ie

- **Stanford Thriving and Surviving** course is a six-week self-management programme, developed by Stanford University, and run by Purple House. It includes information about exercise: www.purplehouse.ie/stanford-cancer-thriving-surviving-programme

Not to be confused with…

- **Survive and Thrive**. Marie Keating Foundation's Survive and Thrive workshops and seminars have been created to help men and women who have finished cancer treatment to adapt to the 'new normal.' These workshops include information about physical activity. www.mariekeating.ie/cancer-services/survive-and-thrive/

References

Introduction

1. National Cancer Institute (2020) *Physical Activity and Cancer*. Available at: www.cancer.gov/about-cancer/causes-prevention/risk/obesity/physical-activity-fact-sheet (Accessed: 18 July 2021).

2. Cormie P, Zopf EM, Zhang X, Schmitz KH. The impact of exercise on cancer mortality, recurrence, and treatment-related adverse effects. *Epidemiologic Reviews* 2017; 39(1): 71–92. https://doi.org/10.1093/epirev/mxx007

3. The Guardian. Cancer: 'If exercise was a pill it would be prescribed to every patient. *The Guardian* 7 May 2018. www.theguardian.com/society/2018/may/07/cancer-if-exercise-was-a-pill-it-would-be-prescribed-to-every-patient (Accessed: 18 July 2021).

4. Cormie P, Atkinson M, Bucci L, Cust A, *et al.* Clinical Oncology Society of Australia position statement on exercise in cancer care. *Med J Aust* 2018; 209(4): 184–187. doi: 10.5694/mja18.00199

5. NHS Manchester (2020) *Prehab4cancer Recovery Programme*. Available at: www.prehab4cancer.co.uk/ (Accessed 11 August 2021).

6. National Cancer Institute (2020) *Physical Activity and Cancer*. Available at: www.cancer.gov/about-cancer/causes-prevention/risk/obesity/physical-activity-fact-sheet (Accessed: 18 July 2021).

7. Salerno EA, Saint-Maurice PF, Willis EA, Moore SC, DiPietro L, Matthews CE. Ambulatory function and mortality among cancer survivors in the NIH-AARP Diet and Health Study. *Cancer Epidemiology Biomarkers & Prevention* 2021; 30(4): 690-698. https://doi.org/10.1158/1055-9965.EPI-20-1473

8. 'Sedentary lifestyle' (2009) *Medical Dictionary*. Available at: https://medical-dictionary.thefreedictionary.com/sedentary+lifestyle (Accessed: 18 July 2021).

9. Berrino, F. Lifestyle prevention of cancer recurrence: the yin and the yang. *Cancer Treat Res* 2014; 159: 341–351. https://pubmed.ncbi.nlm.nih.gov/24114490/

10. Berkovitz, B. (n.d.) *Don't just sit there*. Available at: www.vcccd.edu/sites/default/files/departments/human-resources/professional-development/dontjustsitthere.pdf (Accessed: 18 July 2021).

Chapter 1: How exercise can help with the impact and side effects of cancer treatment

1. Cancer Research UK (2020) *What is cancer fatigue?* Available at: www.cancerresearchuk.org/about-cancer/coping/physically/fatigue/what-is-cancer-fatigue (Accessed: 18 July 2021).
2. Cancer Research UK (2020) *Causes of cancer fatigue*. Available at: https://about-cancer.cancerresearchuk.org/about-cancer/coping/physically/fatigue/causes (Accessed: 18 July 2021).
3. Gladwell VF, Brown DK, Wood C, Sandercock GR, Barton JL. The great outdoors: how a green exercise environment can benefit all. *Extreme Physiology & Medicine* 2013; 2: 3. https://extremephysiolmed.biomedcentral.com/articles/10.1186/2046-7648-2-3
4. Mustian KM, Sprod LK, Janelsins M, Peppone LJ, Mohile S. Exercise recommendations for cancer-related fatigue, cognitive impairment, sleep problems, depression, pain, anxiety, and physical dysfunction: a review. *Oncol Hematol Rev* 2012; 8(2): 81–88. www.ncbi.nlm.nih.gov/pmc/articles/PMC3647480/
5. Dennett AM, Peiris CL, Shields N, Prendergast LA, Taylor NF. Moderate-intensity exercise reduces fatigue and improves mobility in cancer survivors: a systematic review and meta-regression. *Journal of Physiotherapy* 2016; 62(2): 68–82. www.journalofphysiotherapy.com/article/S1836-9553(16)00021-7/fulltext
6. Adams SC, DeLorey DS, Davenport MH, Fairey AS, North S, Courneya KS. Effects of high-intensity interval training on fatigue and quality of life in testicular cancer survivors. *British Journal of Cancer* 2018; 118(10): 1313–1321. https://pubmed.ncbi.nlm.nih.gov/29736007/
7. Mugele H, Freitag N, Wilhemi J, Yang Y, *et al*. High-intensity interval training in the therapy and aftercare of cancer patients: a systematic review with meta-analysis. *Journal Cancer Surviv* 2019; 13(2): 205–223. https://pubmed.ncbi.nlm.nih.gov/30806875/
8. Mustian KM, Sprod LK, Janelsins M, Peppone LJ, Mohile S. Exercise recommendations for cancer-related fatigue, cognitive impairment, sleep problems, depression, pain, anxiety, and physical dysfunction: a review. *Oncol Hematol Rev* 2012; 8(2): 81–88. www.ncbi.nlm.nih.gov/pmc/articles/PMC3647480/
9. Thorneycroft J. (2019) *Mental Health Inequalities and Cancer*, Macmillan Cancer Support. Available at: https://think.macmillan.org.uk/mental-health-inequalities-and-cancer-40afe72df62a (Accessed: 18 July 2021).
10. Mental Health Foundation Scotland (2018) *Cancer patients left to cope with mental health problems alone*. Available at: www.mentalhealth.org.uk/news/cancer-patients-left-cope-mental-health-problems-alone (Accessed: 18 July 2021).
11. Pitman A, Suleman S, Hyde N, Hodgkiss. Depression and anxiety in patients with cancer. *BMJ* 2018; 361: k1415. https://pubmed.ncbi.nlm.nih.gov/29695476/

12. Chekroud SR, Gueorguieva R, Zheutlin AB, Paulus, *et al*. Association between physical exercise and mental health in 1.2 million individuals in the USA between 2011 and 2015: a cross-sectional study. *Lancet Psychiatry* 2018; 5(9): 739–746.
DOI: 10.1016/S2215-0366(18)30227-X https://pubmed.ncbi.nlm.nih.gov/30099000/

13. Fong DYT, Ho JWC, Hui BPH, Lee AM, *et al*. Physical activity for cancer survivors: meta-analysis of randomised controlled trials. *BMJ* 2012; 344: e70.
https://pubmed.ncbi.nlm.nih.gov/22294757/ (Accessed: 18 July 2018).

14. Galvao DA, Newton RU, Chambers SK, Spry N, *et al*. Psychological distress in men with prostate cancer undertaking androgen deprivation therapy: modifying effects of exercise from a year-long randomized controlled trial. *Prostate Cancer and Prostatic Diseases* 15 January 2021. https://doi.org/10.1038/s41391-021-00327-2

15. Levin GT, Greenwood KM, Singh F, *et al*. Exercise improves physical function and mental health of brain cancer survivors: two exploratory case studies. *Integrative Cancer Therapies* 2015; 15(2): 190–196. https://doi.org/10.1177/1534735415600068

16. Johnson S. What is the emotional impact of cancer? Discussion roundup. *The Guardian* 29 May 2014. Available at: www.theguardian.com/society/2014/may/29/cancer-emotional-psychological-impact-discussion-roundup (Accessed: 18 July 2021).

17. Cancer Research UK (2021) *Osteoporosis risk and hormone therapy*. Available at: www.cancerresearchuk.org/about-cancer/cancer-in-general/treatment/hormone-therapy/osteoporosis (Accessed: 18 July 2021).

18. Schwartz A, Winters-Stone K, Gallucci B. Exercise effects on bone mineral density in women with breast cancer receiving adjuvant chemotherapy. *Oncology Nursing Forum* 2007; 34(3): 627-633. doi:10.1188/07.ONF.627-633

19. Almstedt HC, Grote S, Korte JR, Beaudion SP, *et al*. Combined aerobic and resistance training improves bone health of female cancer survivors. *Bone Reports* 2016; 5: 274–279. https://doi.org/10.1016/j.bonr.2016.09.003 www.sciencedirect.com/science/article/pii/S2352187216300389

20. Lee CE, Leslie WD, Czaykowski P, Gingerich J, *et al*. A comprehensive bone-health management approach for men with prostate cancer receiving androgen deprivation therapy. *Curr Oncol* 2011; 18(4): 163–172.
DOI: 10.3747/co.v18i4.746 https://pubmed.ncbi.nlm.nih.gov/21874106/

21. Ferioli M, Zauli G, Martelli AM, Vitale M, *et al*. Impact of physical exercise in cancer survivors during and after antineoplastic treatments. *Oncotarget* 2018; 9(17): 14005–14034.
doi: 10.18632/oncotarget.24456

22. Vance V, Mourtzakis M, McCargar L, Hanning R. Weight gain in breast cancer survivors: prevalence, pattern and health consequences. *Obesity Review* 2011; 12(4): 282–294.
https://doi.org/10.1111/j.1467-789X.2010.00805.x

23. Dawson JK, Dorff TB, Schroeder ET, Lane CJ, *et al*. Impact of resistance training on body composition and metabolic syndrome variables during androgen deprivation therapy for prostate cancer: a pilot randomized controlled trial. *BMC Cancer* 2018; 18(1): 368.
https://bmccancer.biomedcentral.com/articles/10.1186/s12885-018-4306-9

24. Fearon K, Arends J, Baracos V. Understanding the mechanisms and treatment options in cancer cachexia. *Nat Rev Clin Oncol* 2013; 10(2): 90–99. https://pubmed.ncbi.nlm.nih.gov/23207794/

25. Jönsson C, Johansson K. The effects of pole walking on arm lymphoedema and cardiovascular fitness in women treated for breast cancer: a pilot and feasibility study. *Physiotherapy Theory and Practice* 2013; 30(4): 236–242. www.tandfonline.com/doi/abs/10.3109/09593985.2013.848961

26. Buttigliero C, Vana F, Bertaglia V, Vignani, *et al*. The fat body mass increase after adjuvant androgen deprivation therapy is predictive of prostate cancer outcome. *Endocrine* 2015; 50: 223–230. https://link.springer.com/article/10.1007/s12020-015-0525-x

27. Playdon MC, Bracken MB, Sanft TB, Ligibel JA, *et al*. Weight gain after breast cancer diagnosis and all-cause mortality: systematic review and meta-analysis. *J Natl Cancer Inst* 2015; 107(12): djv275. doi: 10.1093/jnci/djv275.

28. ACE (n.d.) *Percent Body Fat Calculator: Skinfold Method*. Available at: www.acefitness.org/education-and-resources/lifestyle/tools-calculators/percent-body-fat-calculator (Accessed: 18 July 2021).

29. Prostate Cancer UK (n.d.) *Men, we are with you*. Available at: www.prostatecanceruk.org (Accessed: 11 August 2021).

30. Lymphoedema Support Network (n.d.) *Exercise and movement*. Available at: www.lymphoedema.org/information/useful-articles/exercise-and-movement (Accessed: 8 August 2021)

31. Jönsson C, Johansson K. The effects of pole walking on arm lymphoedema and cardiovascular fitness in women treated for breast cancer: a pilot and feasibility study', *Physiotherapy Theory and Practice* 2013; 30(4): 236–242. www.tandfonline.com/doi/abs/10.3109/09593985.2013.848961

32. Di Blasio A, Morano T, Napolitano G, Bucci I, *et al*. Nordic walking and the Isa method for breast cancer survivors: effects on upper limb circumferences and total body extracellular water – a pilot study. *Breast Care* 2016; 11(6): 428-431. DOI: 10.1159/000453599 https://pubmed.ncbi.nlm.nih.gov/28228712/

33. Schmitz KH, Ahmed RL, Troxel AB, Cheville A, *et al*. Weight lifting for women at risk for breast cancer-related lymphoedema: a randomized trial. *JAMA 2010;* 304(24): 2699–2705. doi:10.1001/jama.2010.1837

34. Nelson NL. Breast cancer–Related lymphedema and resistance exercise: a systematic review. *Journal of Strength and Conditioning Research* 2016; 30(9): 2656–2665. doi: 10.1519/JSC.0000000000001355

35. Loudon A, Barnett T, Williams A. Yoga, breast cancer-related lymphoedema and well-being: a descriptive report of women's participation in a clinical trial. *J Clin Nurs* 2017; 26(23-24): 4685–4695. https://pubmed.ncbi.nlm.nih.gov/28334470/

36. Avancini A, *et al*. Exercise prehabilitation in lung cancer: getting stronger to recover faster. *European Journal of Surgical Oncology* 2021; 47(8): 1847–1855. www.sciencedirect.com/science/article/abs/pii/S0748798321003723

37. Howley EK. Should I exercise with lung cancer? *US News* 15 October 2018. Available at: https://health.usnews.com/health-care/patient-advice/articles/2018-10-15/should-i-exercise-with-lung-cancer (Accessed: 18 July 2021).

38. Peddle-McIntyre CJ, Singh F, Thomas R, Newton RU, *et al*. Exercise training for advanced lung cancer. *Cochrane Database of Systematic Reviews* 2019; 2: Art No: CD012685. DOI: 10.1002/14651858.CD012685.pub2..

39. Roy Castle Lung Cancer Foundation (n.d.) *Getting active and exercising*. Available at: https://roycastle.org/about-lung-cancer/living-with-lung-cancer/getting-active/ (Accessed: 18 July 2021).

40. The West Way to Swim (n.d.) *Stretching exercises to improve breathing, lung function and buoyancy*. Available at: www.swim-west.com/stretching-exercises-to-improve-breathing-lung-function-and-buoyancy/ (Accessed: 18 July 2021).

41. Bladder & Bowel Community (2021) *What Is A Stoma?* Available at: www.bladderandbowel.org/bowel/stoma/what-is-a-stoma/ (Accessed: 18 July 2021).

42. Russell S (2020) *The Bowel Cancer Recovery Toolkit*. London: Hammersmith Books. Available at: https://www.hammersmithbooks.co.uk/product/the-bowel-cancer-recovery-toolkit/ (Accessed: 18 July 2021).

43. Colostomy UK (2019) *What is a parastomal hernia?* Available at: www.colostomyuk.org/information/stoma-problems/parastomalhernia/ (Accessed: 18 July 2021).

44. Colostomy UK (2019) *Top Tips For Being Active*. Available at: www.colostomyuk.org/category/top-tips-for-being-active/ (Accessed: 18 July 2021).

45. Cancer.Net (2021) *Urinary Incontinence*. Available at: www.cancer.net/coping-with-cancer/physical-emotional-and-social-effects-cancer/managing-physical-side-effects/urinary-incontinence (Accessed: 18 July 2021).

46. Macmillan Cancer Support (2018) *Macmillan toilet card*. Available at: https://be.macmillan.org.uk/be/p-24952-macmillan-toilet-card.aspx (Accessed: 8 August 2021).

47. Breastcancer.org (2020) *Exercise after surgery*. Available at: www.breastcancer.org/tips/exercise/treatment/surgery (Accessed: 8 August 2021).

48. Breast Cancer Research UK (2021) *Breast reconstruction*. Available at: www.cancerresearchuk.org/about-cancer/breast-cancer/treatment/surgery/breast-reconstruction (Accessed: 8 August 2021).

49. Science Direct (n.d.) *Chemotherapy-induced peripheral neuropathy*. Available at: www.sciencedirect.com/topics/medicine-and-dentistry/chemotherapy-induced-peripheral-neuropathy (Accessed: 18 July 2021).

50. Wonders KY, Drury DG. Current exercise behaviors of breast cancer patients diagnosed with chemotherapy-induced peripheral neuropathy. *Journal of Integrative Oncology* 2012; 1: 103. www.hilarispublisher.com/abstract/current-exercise-behaviors-of-breast-cancer-patients-diagnosed-with-chemotherapyinduced-peripheral-neuropathy-25214.html

51. Wonders KY. The effect of supervised exercise training on symptoms of chemotherapy induced peripheral neuropathy. *Int J Phys Med Rehabil* 2014; 2: 4. www.scholarscentral.com/abstract/the-effect-of-supervised-exercise-training-on-symptoms-of-chemotherapyinduced-peripheral-neuropathy-34053.html

52. Wikipedia (n.d.) *Chemotherapy-induced peripheral neuropathy*. Available at: https://en.wikipedia.org/wiki/Chemotherapy-induced_peripheral_neuropathy#Other_therapeutics (Accessed: 18 July 2021).

53. Galantino ML, Brooks J, Tiger R, Jang S, Wilson K. Effectiveness of somatic yoga and meditation: a pilot study in a multicultural cancer survivor population with chemotherapy-induced peripheral neuropathy. *Int J Yoga Therapy* 2020; 30(1): 49-61. DOI: 10.17761/2020-D-18-00030 https://pubmed.ncbi.nlm.nih.gov/31483689/

Chapter 2: When – the different phases of cancer

1. Macmillan Cancer Support (n.d.) *Prehabilitation for People with Cancer*. Available at: https://cdn.macmillan.org.uk/dfsmedia/1a6f23537f7f4519bb0cf14c45b2a629/1532-10061/options/download/prehabilitation-for-people-with-cancer-tcm9-353994 (Accessed: 18 July 2021).

2. BBC News. Wrexham 'prehabilitation' programme helps patients get in shape. *BBC News* 28 November 2019. Available at: www.bbc.co.uk/news/uk-wales-50575808 (Accessed: 18 July 2021).

3. Macmillan Cancer Support (n.d.) *Prehabilitation for People with Cancer*. Available at: https://cdn.macmillan.org.uk/dfsmedia/1a6f23537f7f4519bb0cf14c45b2a629/1532-10061/options/download/prehabilitation-for-people-with-cancer-tcm9-353994 (Accessed: 18 July 2021).

4. Moore J, Merchant Z, Rowlinson K, McEwan K, Evison M, Faulkner G, Sultan J, McPhee JS, Steele J. Implementing a system-wide cancer prehabilitation programme: The journey of Greater Manchester's 'Prehab4cancer'. *European Journal of Surgical Oncology* 2020; 47(3): 524-532. https://doi.org/10.1016/j.ejso.2020.04.042

5. Cancer Research UK (2019) *Exercise guidelines for cancer patients*. Available at: www.cancerresearchuk.org/about-cancer/coping/physically/exercise-guidelines (Accessed: 18 July 2021).

6. BloodCancer.com (2018) *Watchful Waiting*. Available at: https://blood-cancer.com/treatment/watch-wait/(Accessed: 18 July 2021).

7. Thomas VJ, Seet-Lee C, Marthick M, Cheema BS, *et al*. Aerobic exercise during chemotherapy infusion for cancer treatment: a novel randomised crossover safety and feasibility trial. *Support Care Cancer 2020;* 28(2): 625–632. https://link.springer.com/article/10.1007/s00520-019-04871-5

8. Adamsen L, Quist M, Andersen C, Moller T, *et al*. Effect of a multimodal high intensity exercise intervention in cancer patients undergoing chemotherapy: randomised controlled trial. *BMJ* 2009; 339: b3410. doi: 10.1136/bmj.b3410 https://pubmed.ncbi.nlm.nih.gov/?term=Adamsen+L&cauthor_id=19826172 (Accessed: 18 July 2021).

9. McLaughlin M, Christie A, Campbell A. Case report of exercise to attenuate side effects of treatment for pancreatic cancer. *Case Rep Oncol* 2019; 12(3): 845-854. • DOI:10.1159/000503815

10. Windsor PM, Nicol KF, Potter J. A randomized, controlled trial of aerobic exercise for treatment-related fatigue in men receiving radical external beam radiotherapy for localized prostate carcinoma. *Cancer* 2004; 101(3). https://acsjournals.onlinelibrary.wiley.com/action/doSearch?ContribAuthorStored=Windsor%2C+Phyllis+M (Accessed: 18 July 2021).

11. Piraux E, Caty G, Nana FA, Reychler. Effects of exercise therapy in cancer patients undergoing radiotherapy treatment: a narrative review. *Sage Open Medicine* 2020; 8: 1-21. https://journals.sagepub.com/doi/full/10.1177/2050312120922657

12. Hyatt A, Drosdowsky A, Williams N. Exercise behaviors and fatigue in patients receiving immunotherapy for advanced melanoma: a cross-sectional survey via social media. *Integrated Cancer Therapy* 2019; 8: 1-9. https://doi.org/10.1177/1534735419864431

13. McNeeley ML, Peddle CJ, Parliament M, Courneya KS. Cancer rehabilitation: recommendations for integrating exercise programming in the clinical practice setting. *Current Cancer Therapy Reviews* 2006; 2(4): 351-360. DOI: 10.2174/157339406778699187 www.eurekaselect.com/58071/article

14. Macmillan Cancer Support (2012) *The importance of physical activity for people living with and beyond cancer.* Available at: https://be.macmillan.org.uk/Downloads/CancerInformation/LivingWithAndAfterCancer/MAC138200415PhysicalActivityevidencereviewDIGITAL.pdf (Accessed: 8 August 2021).

15. Wilk M, Kepski J, Kepska J, Casselli S, Szmit S. Exercise interventions in metastatic cancer disease: a literature review and a brief discussion on current and future perspectives. *BMJ Supportive & Palliative Care 2020;* 10: 404–410. http://dx.doi.org/10.1136/bmjspcare-2020-002487 https://spcare.bmj.com/content/10/4/404

16. Macmillan Cancer Support (n.d.) *Physical activity for people with metastatic bone disease – Guidance for professionals.* Available at: https://cdn.macmillan.org.uk/dfsmedia/1a6f23537f7f4519bb0cf14c45b2a629/1784-source/physical-activity-for-people-with-metastatic-bone-disease-guidance-tcm9-326004?_ga=2.195379108.98154908.1612357246-904080291.1612357246 (Accessed: 18 July 2021).

17. Mental Health Foundation Scotland (2018) *Cancer patients left to cope with mental health problems alone.* Available at: www.mentalhealth.org.uk/news/cancer-patients-left-cope-mental-health-problems-alone (Accessed: 18 July 2021).

18. Goodheart F, Atkins L. *The Cancer Survivor's Companion: Practical Ways to Cope with your Feelings after Cancer.* London, UK: Piatkus; 2011.

19. Becker R. Palliative care 1: principles of palliative care nursing and end-of-life care. *Nursing Times* 2009; 105: 13. www.nursingtimes.net/clinical-archive/end-of-life-and-palliative-care/palliative-care-1-principles-of-palliative-care-nursing-and-end-of-life-care-07-04-2009

20. Cancer Exercise Toolkit (n.d.) *Advanced Cancer and Palliative Care*. Available at: https://cancerexercisetoolkit.trekeducation.org/screening-and-safety/special-populations/specific-cancer-streams/advanced-cancer/ (Accessed: 18 July 2021).
21. Turner K. (2016) *Promoting wellbeing through exercise in our hospices*. Available at: www.mariecurie.org.uk/blog/exercise-wellbeing-hospices/56379 (Accessed: 18 July 2021).
22. Kowalski SL. Physical therapy and exercise for hospice patients. *Home Healthcare Now* 2016; 34(10): 563–568. https://journals.lww.com/homehealthcarenurseonline/toc/2016/11000 (Accessed: 18 July 2021).

Chapter 3: What to do, and how

1. Cancer Research UK (2020) *What is cancer fatigue?* Available at: www.cancerresearchuk.org/about-cancer/coping/physically/fatigue/what-is-cancer-fatigue (Accessed: 19 July 2021).
2. Mustian K, Sprod LK, Janelsins M, Peppone LJ, Mohile S. Exercise recommendations for cancer-related fatigue, cognitive impairment, sleep problems, depression, pain, anxiety, and physical dysfunction: a review. *Oncol Hematol Rev* 2012; 8(2): 81–88. www.ncbi.nlm.nih.gov/pmc/articles/PMC3647480/
3. Gotink RA, Hermans KSFM, Gescwind N, De Nooji R, *et al.* Mindfulness and mood stimulate each other in an upward spiral: a mindful walking intervention using experience sampling. *Mindfulness* 2016; 7(5): 1114–1122. www.ncbi.nlm.nih.gov/pmc/articles/PMC5010615/ (Accessed: 19 July 2021).
4. BorrowMyDoggy (2021) Available at: www.borrowmydoggy.com (Accessed: 19 July 2021).
5. MacMillan A. (2017) It's official: dog owners walk way more. *Health.com*. Available at: www.health.com/pets/dog-owners-walk-more-moderate-exercise (Accessed: 19 July 2021).
6. Gov.UK (2020) *UK Chief Medical Officers' Physical Activity Guidelines*. London: Department of Health and Social Care. Available at: www.gov.uk/government/publications/physical-activity-guidelines-uk-chief-medical-officers-report (Accessed: 19 July 2021).
7. Ali C (n.d.) How to work 'exercise snacks' into your day. *Beyond* (University of British Columbia). Available at: https://beyond.ubc.ca/exercise-snacks/ (Accessed: 19 July 2021).
8. Schmitz KH, Courneya KS, Matthews C, Demark-Wahnefried W, *et al.* American College of Sports Medicine roundtable on exercise guidelines for cancer survivors. *Med & Sci in Sports & Exerc* 2010; 42(7): 1409–1426. doi: 10.1249/MSS.0b013e3181e0c112
9. Wonders KY, Stout B, Ondreka D. A model approach to group exercise in cancer survivors. *Phys Med Rehabil Res 1* 2016. doi: 10.15761/PMRR.1000102
10. Galvão DA, Chambers SK. Exercise medicine in men with prostate cancer: breaking barriers to increase participation. *Prostate Cancer and Prostatic Diseases* 2021. www.nature.com/articles/s41391-021-00406-4
11. Campbell KL, Winters-Stone KM, Wiskemann J, May AM, *et al.* Exercise guidelines for cancer survivors: consensus statement from International Multidisciplinary Roundtable. *Med Sci Sports & Exercise* 2019; 51(11): 2375–2390. DOI: 10.1249/MSS.0000000000002116 https://pubmed.ncbi.nlm.nih.gov/31626055/

12. Kato T, Tomioka T, Yamashita T, Yamamoto H, *et al.* Nordic walking increases distal radius bone mineral content in young women. *J Sports Sci Med* 2020; 19(2): 237–244. https://pubmed.ncbi.nlm.nih.gov/?term=Kato+T&cauthor_id=32390716

13. DiBlasio A, Morano T, Bucci I, DiSanto S, *et al.* Physical exercises for breast cancer survivors: effects of 10 weeks of training on upper limb circumferences. *J Phys Ther Sci* 2016; 28: 2778–2784. www.jstage.jst.go.jp/article/jpts/28/10/28_JPTS-2016-375/_pdf/-char/en

14. Fischer M, Krol-Warmerdam EMM, Ranke GMC, Vermeulen HM, et al. Stick Together: A Nordic Walking Group Intervention for Breast Cancer Survivors. *J Psychosoc Oncol* 2015; 33(3): 278-296.
www.ncbi.nlm.nih.gov/pubmed/25751587 www.ncbi.nlm.nih.gov/pubmed/25751587

15. Boutcher SH. High-intensity intermittent exercise and fat loss. *Journal of Obesity* 2011; 2011: Article ID 868305. doi: 10.1155/2011/868305

16. Mugele H, Freitag N, Wilhelmi J, Yang Y, *et al.* High-intensity interval training in the therapy and aftercare of cancer patients: a systematic review with meta-analysis. *Journal Cancer Surviv* 2019; 13(2): 205–223. https://pubmed.ncbi.nlm.nih.gov/30806875/ (Accessed: 18 July 2021).

17. Nursing Times. Is exercise to blame for Andrew Marr's stroke? *Nursing Times* 23 April 2013. www.nursingtimes.net/news/behind-the-headlines/is-exercise-to-blame-for-andrew-marrs-stroke-23-04-2013/ (Accessed: 19 July 2021).

18. Parkrun (2021) Available at: www.parkrun.com/about (Accessed: 19 July 2021).

19. Craft LL, Perna FM. The benefits of exercise for the clinically depressed. *J Clinical Psychiatry* 2004; 6(3): 104–111. www.ncbi.nlm.nih.gov/pmc/articles/PMC474733/

20. Anxiety & Depression Association of America (2021) *Exercise for stress and anxiety.* Available at: https://adaa.org/living-with-anxiety/managing-anxiety/exercise-stress-and-anxiety (Accessed: 19 July 2021).

21. Razmus A. (2019) The role of gratitude in sports performance. *Competitive Edge Physical Therapy.* Available at: www.compedgept.com/blog/gratitude-and-sports-performance (Accessed: 19 July 2021).

22. Dupuy O, Douzi W, Theurot D, Bosquet L, Dugue B. An evidence-based approach for choosing post-exercise recovery techniques to reduce markers of muscle damage, soreness, fatigue, and inflammation: A systematic review with meta-analysis. *Front Physiol* 2018; 9: 403. doi:10.3389/fphys.2018.00403

23. NHS (2020) *Treatment: sports injuries.* Available at: www.nhs.uk/conditions/sports-injuries/treatment/ (Accessed: 19 July 2021).

Chapter 4: The practical section

1. Diep C Foundation (2019) *Basic Core Strengthening Exercises Pre & Post Breast Reconstruction Surgery.* https://youtu.be/xriMg6Yde-l

Index

Note: Illustrations (figures and tables) are comprehensively referred to from the text (usually on same or following page). Illustrations have only been given a page reference in the absence of their concomitant mention in the text referring to that illustration.

**Also from Hammersmith
Health Books**

The Bowel Cancer
Recovery Toolkit

By Sarah Russell

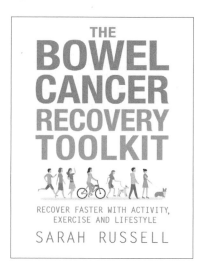

A practical guide to exercising before and after abdominal surgery, especially for cancer, looking at what is safe and effective and what other lifestyle strategies will work with movement and exercise to mitigate the effects of cancer treatment and lower the risk of recurrence.

'Sarah's book is a fantastic starting point for someone living with or beyond colorectal cancer who wants to find out more about exercise during and after cancer treatment. Being active is one of the biggest things you can do to improve your experience and this book will help you achieve that.'

Dr Lucy Gossage, oncologist, triathlete, editor of www.cancerfit.me